Commercial Broiler Chicken Production

Commercial Broiler Chicken Production

Dr. M.MURUGAN, M.V.Sc., Ph.D., M.B.A.,
Associate Professor
Department of Livestock Products Technology
Veterinary College and Research Institute
Tirunelveli, Tamil Nadu - 627 358
Email: mailstommurugan@gmail.com

SSPH

SATISH SERIAL PUBLISHING HOUSE
403, Express Tower, Commercial Complex
Azadpur, Delhi-110033 (India)
Telefax : 011 - 47073040
e-mail : info@satishserial.com, hkjain1975@yahoo.com
Website : www.satishserial.com

Published by :

SATISH SERIAL PUBLISHING HOUSE

403, Express Tower, Commercial Complex, Azadpur, Delhi-110033 (India)
Telefax : 011 - 47073040
E-mail : info@satishserial.com, hkjain1975@yahoo.com

Print Again, 2025

ISBN 978-93-85055-90-4

Composed, Designed & Printed in India

Preface

Commercial broiler chicken production is a vibrant farming entity in commercial poultry farming sector of India, and witnessing the annual growth rate of 6-8 per cent. The production system of commercial broiler chicken is highly scientific and characterized by intensive farming systems as high input - high output production mode.

Though, there are few text books available on commercial broiler production, there is a long felt need exists for a scientific, comprehensive, practical oriented book on commercial broiler chicken production with special reference to Indian farming conditions. Considering that, this book is planned to cater the needs of veterinary technocrats, broiler farm managers, farming aspirants, students of veterinary science, in terms of acting as handy book for their use in application of scientific farming principles in their regular professional practice.

In this book, the subject matter has been arranged in a sequential manner for easy understanding of the concepts and its way of application through activities at the end of each chapter. I strongly encourage the student readers to practice the exercises for better understanding and to gain confidence during execution.

I put forth my sincere thanks to Satish Serial Publishing House for publishing and promoting this book in an attractive manner.

Finally, I express my loveable thanks to my wife *Abbi* and my *daughters Muthamil and Manicka* for encouraging me to write this book.

Date: 23.05.2016 **M. Murugan**
Place: Tirunelveli - 627 358

Contents

Chapter 1

History of Broiler Chicken Production in India

Learning objectives:

1. *Know the historical perspectives of broiler chicken farming in India*
2. *Discuss the current status of commercial broiler chicken farming in India*

Brief history of commercial broiler production in India

The term, Poultry, comprises of all domesticated species of birds used in commercial rearing for food and other economic purposes, which includes chicken, duck, turkey, Japanese quail, guinea fowl and, ratites such as ostrich and emu. However, commercial poultry production of India mainly revolves around farming activities such as broiler chicken farms, layer chicken farms for chicken meat and egg production.

In India, the Christian missionaries were the first to start commercial poultry farming, towards the beginning of the twentieth century. The first Christian mission poultry farm was established in Etah, Uttar Pradesh state of India in 1912 and the first poultry exhibition was held at Lucknow in 1912.

The period of third and fourth five year plans (1961-1974) was actually the turning point in the development of poultry industry in the country. Intensive Poultry Development Programme was introduced in Third Five Year Plan (1961-1966) to provide all the essential inputs like improved genetic stocks and farm advisory services to farmers in the form of a package.

Generally, the term, Broiler, indicates the young, immature, fast growing chicken stock of either sex, usually slaughtered at 5-7 weeks of age, with the live weight of 2-3 kg. It is a soft, tender, juicy white meat with pliable skin, flexible breast bone cartilage and low separable fat.

The commercial broiler production of India is around 50 years old and considering history of domestication of chicken, it is very recent in origin. The humble start of broiler production was first taken place at Andhra Pradesh state of India in 1959 by importing White Rock and Cornish chicks from Israel.

Central government institutions like regional Central Poultry Development Organizations (CPDO), All India Coordinated Research Projects on Chicken meat of Indian Council of Agricultural Research (ICAR), New Delhi, Central Avian Research Institute (CARI) of Bareilly, Uttar Pradesh, and state agricultural and veterinary universities are the key organizations involved in popularising, promoting and scientific development of broiler industry in India.

The role of private players/breeding companies in broiler production started during early seventies by importing improved genetic stocks from foreign countries and establishing own pure line breeding companies in India.

Current status of Indian broiler industry

Indian broiler industry is one the classical success story in India's primary sector production systems. When, growth of agriculture is around 3-4 per cent annually, Indian broiler industry is witnessing a spectacular annual growth of 6-8 per cent. The world's leading broiler chicken producers are United States of America, China, Brazil, European Union, Mexico and India; India stands on sixth position in broiler production with the production of 3.24 million tonnes broiler meat in 2014. However, considering the population of India, the per capita consumption of broiler meat in India is 2.3 kg, which is very low when compared to world per capita consumption of 13.16 kg.

Broiler production and Per capita consumption of broiler meat in India

Year	Broiler meat production (million metric tonnes)	Per capita Consumption (kg)
1961	0.078	0.17
1971	0.095	0.17
1981	0.141	0.20
1991	0.389	0.45
2001	1.07	1.26
2010	2.64	1.90
2011	2.88	2.00
2012	3.06	2.10
2013	3.15	2.20
2014	3.24	2.30

Today, Indian broiler production is highly organized, with the sector contribution of nearly 85 percent of the total output. According to industry sources, approximately 60 to 65 percent of the organized sector is *integrated,* with the remainder operating as independent producers. The production performances of Indian broiler industry are on par with international standards, and India is becoming a hub of broiler chicken production for tropics of the world. The industry is concentrated mainly in Southern states of India, Andhra Pradesh, Tamil Nadu, Karnataka, Maharashtra and West Bengal of East and Haryana of North India.

The driving factors for impressive development of Indian broiler industry are,

1. Income growth of individuals,
2. Comparatively low costing of meat,
3. Rapid urbanization and changing food style,
4. Scientific system of rearing and vertical integration,
5. Competitive production costs,
6. No religious taboo on chicken meat consumption.

However, even with highly organized production system, organized broiler processing and retailing are limited in industry. As per the industry sources, live birds markets make up more than 90 percent of total broilers sales with processed product making up the remainder.

Challenges for commercial broiler production in India

Though, Indian broiler industry is witnessing a spectacular growth trend annually, it is also facing few serious problems like any other agriculture industry like high volatility of markets, instability in pricing, escalating feed costs, welfare and concern about food safety issues etc.

Better understanding about the production system will help the stakeholders to address these issues and application of Good Husbandry Practices (GHP) in broiler production will help to overcome these issues with tangible benefits.

Activity

1. Collect the year wise data on human population and broiler chicken production of your state and work out the per capita consumption and graphically represent the growth trend of the same.
2. Collect the data on leading countries of broiler chicken production and compare the production trends.
3. Compare the per capita consumption of broiler chicken meat of various states of India and offer your comments.

❑❑❑

Chapter 2

Chicken Stocks of Commercial Broiler Production

Learning objectives:

1. *Know about the genetic stocks used in broiler chicken farming*
2. *Discuss about the industrial breeding programme in broiler chicken farming*

Chicken stocks of commercial broiler production are basically "hybrids", which means, the stocks are expressing "hybrid vigour" in their performances. The hybrid vigour of these birds is achieved through systematic selection and cross breeding programme for considerably a long period. In true sense, the commercial broilers are genetically superior (not genetically modified) birds, selected and bred for high and fast growth.

The genetic base for most of the commercial broilers is derived from three classical base breeds namely, Cornish of English origin, New Hampshire and Plymouth Rock of American origin. Initially, the classical plant breeding principles of Hybridization in corn were used for the early development of pure lines, exclusively for sire and dam lines. In most of the sire lines, Cornish breed was used exclusively and as dam lines New Hampshire and Plymouth were used. The generalized industrial breeding programme for broiler stock production is presented below.

Theoretical plan in industrial broiler breeding programme

1. Pure line breeding with pedigreed population
2. Formation of inbred lines (exclusive sire and dam lines)
3. Use and testing of general and specific combining ability between lines
4. Selection of *niking* (combining) lines

5. Crossing of inbred lines – To exploit heterosis or hybrid vigor
6. Supply of unisex (male or female) progeny at grandparent level from great grand parent
7. Crossing of four lines of grandparent to develop parent breeders of male and female to be a two way cross
8. Crossing of parent to form commercial bird to be a four way cross

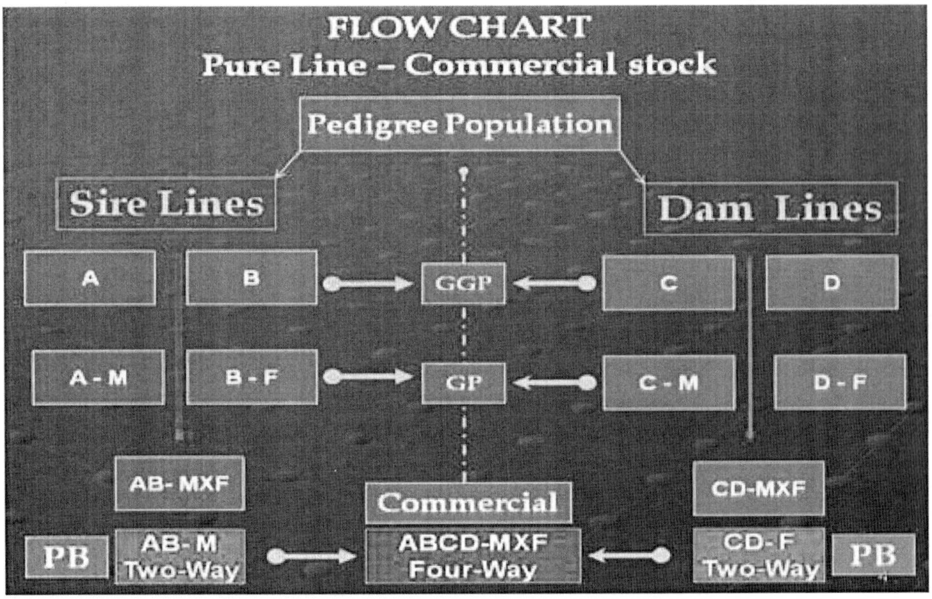

General breeding protocol of industrial broiler breeding

Based on the above programme, it is evident that parent and commercial broiler is two way and four way crosses, which is bestowed with hybrid vigour due to the inbred line crosses in the selection and breeding history of its formation.

Traits of selection

Selection process in broiler breeding is complex, because the stock should be selected for negatively correlated traits. For example, the sire should be selected for high and fast growth with, reasonable fertility and hatchability. The dam should be selected for optimum growth and, good egg production. Since, the high growth in terms of body weight, having negative correlation with fitness traits like egg production and fertility, the selection strategies and breeding plan is becoming complex. However, critical traits of broiler breeding like body weight, egg weight, and rate of weight gain are high to moderately heritable traits. These traits will respond well for individual selection or mass selection. Based on these, breeding programme for male mainly employs the mass selection with considerably large population to maintain the variance for selection. In female lines, mostly family selection or combined selection can be practiced based on the trait in question.

The critical traits for selection in broiler breeding are as follows,

Critical Traits	Minor Traits
1. Growth (Body Weight)	1. Ascites resistance
2. Feed conversion	2. Disease resistance
3. Egg Production	3. Eviscerated Yield
4. Sexual maturity	4. Breast Meat Yield
5. Egg size	5. Breast Conformation
6. Fertility	6. Carcass Leanness
7. Hatchability	7. Condemnation
8. Livability and	8. Carcass uniformity
9. Leg and skeletal strength	

Understanding the superiority of this broiler chicken stock is highly essential, to plan and execute the management programme. These birds have to be supported by good quality housing, feeding and health management progammes, otherwise desirable results cannot be achieved.

The major industrial broiler chicken commercial stocks available in India are :

1. Vencobb
2. Hubbard
3. Hybro
4. Ross
5. Lohmann

The average performance of broiler chicken in Indian farming conditions

1. Market age	42 days
2. Market weight	2.2 kg
3. Feed Efficiency	1.70
4. Livability	95 per cent
5. Performance Efficiency Factor	300 -320
6. Dressing yield	75 per cent

Here, it is always better to know that, individual primary breeding companies recommend their own management and feeding standards for their commercial strains, in which mild variation exists between commercial strain performances and their management specifications. However, understanding the basics of this variation will help the practioners to devise specific plan for a commercial strain in question.

Activity

1. Collect the breed characteristics of classical broiler base breeds of Cornish, New Hampshire and Barred Plymouth Rock.
2. Visit the websites of leading primary poultry breeding companies and collect the broiler strains available for various markets.
3. Compare the production performances of various commercial broiler strains available in India in terms of market weight, market age, feed efficiency, livability and dressing yield.

❑❑❑

Chapter 3

Broiler Farm Planning

Learning objectives:

1. *Describe the various types of planning to start a broiler farm*
2. *Compute the broiler farm area requirement for a commercial broiler farm*

Planning a commercial broiler farm

The starting point of commercial broiler production is planning for the farming system and it is a prerequisite for effective implementation. Broiler farm planning can be classified in to three namely,

1. Venture type plan
2. Farm size and area plan
3. Financial plan

The planning on the above areas will give an overall blueprint of the broiler production activities to be carried out with a time line.

Venture type plan

In India there are two types broiler farming ventures are available for the entrepreneur to choose and they are,

1. Independent broiler farm (own farm)
2. Contract broiler grower farm (integrated farm)

Independent broiler farm

Independent broiler farm is a farm in which, the entrepreneur or promoter or farmer is the full fledged owner of the farm. He has to take care of all the activities of the farm, starts from construction of broiler houses, purchase of chicks and feed, growing process, health cover and marketing. The promoter has to invest money for the all the activities. Large players will prepare their own feed and small farmers of this type will purchase the feed from feed mill operators, which will reduce the profit margin to some extent. Though own marketing through retail mode provides better profits to the farmers, at times of market depression, there is every chance to face considerable loss also. In early eighties, and up to mid nineties, this is the common mode of venturing in broiler farm business in India. The advantages are being the full right owner on the enterprise and better profits and, disadvantage is the unexpected market risks in marketing and high capital investment. This type of broiler farming system is functioning in 20 -25 per cent of industry volume in India even now.

Contract broiler grower farm

In this system, integrator is a big broiler production operator, who performs all the activities of broiler production from breeder management, production of hatching egg and chicks, feed, health cover, technical advices, processing plant and marketing of live and dressed broilers.

Contract broiler farmer is a franchisee of the integrator, for broiler growing process, and integrator will provide all the inputs from chick, feed, health cover and marketing etc. and contract grower will be paid for the services of growing as per the live weight output and efficiency of production. The investment for broiler house, electricity and labour for broiler growing will be borne by contract grower by making a type of agreement. The nature of contract growing of broilers can be summarized as follows,

Contract growing in broiler industry

Contract broiler grower	Integrator
1. Owning of the land	1. Owning parent stocks
2. Establishment of broiler farm and house	2. Owning Hatcheries
3. Purchase of equipment	3. Supply of day old broiler chicks
4. Rearing of broilers with own or hired labour	4. Supply of broiler feed
5. Bering of electricity and litter material cost	5. Supply of medicines and vaccines

6. Getting the growing cost from the integrator for the total live broiler output considering the efficiency as weightage factor	6. Technical advisory services
7. Sale of manure and empty feed bags	7. Pays the farmers for rearing cost, and incentives from profits
8. Repayment of bank finance for broiler house and equipments for a fixed period	8. Market the broilers as per their wish and mostly through traders/ own processing plants

**Almost all large integrators have their own breeding operations, hatcheries, feed mills, processing plants to minimize the production cost*

This system of broiler farm venturing, keep low risks to the contract growers due to market instability and at the same time offer low profit margins to the growers. On the other hand, integrators are investing more on this system of venturing and earning more profits by facing high risk. Moreover, vertical integration offers the possibility of minimizing the overall cost of production and ensures scientific rearing strategies in broiler chicken production. It also benefits the cost economics of business activity by increasing the volume of production, comparatively with low investment. Since the farmer is facing less risk in this system, it is highly suitable for beginners of broiler production.

Moreover, the advantage is that there are no intermediaries: only integrator–farmer–wholesaler in the market. Farmers do not have to make any investments in working capital. There is also risk insurance to farmers from fluctuations in selling process–they get a fixed income. This arrangement has encouraged a number of small farmers to enter in to the broiler business, in order to supplement their income with a stable return on their investment.

Broiler integration has been expanding rapidly in the states of Western and Southern India, Tamil Nadu, Andhra Pradesh, Karnataka and Maharashtra. Now, the practice of this system is slowly moving to the Northern and Eastern parts of India also.

It is strongly advisable to keep retail outlet by independent broiler farmer to offset market vagaries in price of broilers. If he wishes to establish a broiler farm under contract with an integrator, he should know trust worthiness of integrator, the cost of the inputs, and compare this with the rearing cost paid by the integrator to assess the viability of project and recovery of investment.

He should make sure that the integrator will place chicks without undue breaks by making proper agreements. The farmer is advised to consult an experienced qualified poultry consultant for other technical details, and also to visit a few successful broiler farmers in their area to get the first hand experience.

1. Farm area and layout plan

The entrepreneur, who wishes to start a broiler farm business, has to first assess the market potential of the area, as well as the average market price. Once the decision on the type of venturing is finalized, decision on the size of the farm is playing a crucial role for profitability of the business.

In India, effective and minimum economic farm size for broilers is 5000 -10,000 for independent farm and 10,000 to 20,000 for contract grower farm. The promoter has to make his choices in accordance with the finance capability. The availability of various inputs, like quality chicks, feed, medicines, vaccines, litter material, labour, etc., has to be assessed. After-sale technical and marketing services by the chick and feed suppliers have to be checked.

Identification and selection of farm site

Identification and selection of ideal broiler farm site is a serious process, which involves a number of activities, and needs careful application of mind for the successful functioning of the project. In this process, selection of wrong site will be a permanent problem and it will be a pre disposing factor for other managemental problems.

Identification and selection of farm site starts from the point of making decision on the farm size in broiler farming. It depends on two critical factors like capital input and marketability of the meat output. Once we decide the size of the farm, we can decide on the farm area and other parameters like topography, availability of utilities and inputs, access to logistics and environmental regulations of the area in question.

How to decide the farm area requirement?

A broiler farm layout will have two components and they are called as Build up area (broiler Houses and accessory facilities like feed mills, workers quarters, office, sales counter, godown etc.,) and

Non build up area (vacant land between two broiler houses and other vacant land around the farm). Build up area in any farm is depends on flock size (number of birds to be reared), floor space requirements, and area requirements for other facilities like feed mill, labour quarters, water tank, retail outlet if any etc., Non build up area mainly consists of vacant land, that is distance between two broiler houses, vacant land for future expansions etc.,

2. Construction Co-efficient

Construction Co efficient is a tool will be useful to arrive the farm area requirement for a given farm size. It is defined as the *Ratio of build up area to the total farm area* and calculated as follows,

Construction Co efficient = Build up area / Total farm area

The ideal construction co efficient for smaller farm size operations (up to 30,000 broilers) is 0.40 - 0.50 and, for larger farm operations it should be maximum of 0.30. Considering the construction coefficient, we can also calculate the total farm area requirement for a farm size

Example: 1

A broiler farm with 100,000 sq.ft total area and 35,000 sq.ft build up area will have the construction co efficient of 0.35 (35,000/ 1, 00,000 = 0.35).

Example: 2

A broiler farm with 15,000 sq.ft build up area will be required 50,000 sq.ft total farm area for smooth functioning of the project and future expansions, with the construction co efficient of 0.30.

1. Build up area / Total farm area = Construction Co efficient
2. 15,000 / Total farm area (X) = 0.30
3. Total farm area (X) = Build up area (15,000) / Construction Co efficient (0.30)
4. Total farm area requirement : 15000 / 0.30 = 50,000 sq.ft

How to select a farm site?

In farm site selection, a number of factors have to be considered to design a good farm layout, smooth flow of input and output logistics and to keep a strict bio security programme for disease prevention. Following are the indicative list of factors for consideration.

1. **Topography:** The farm site soil should be virgin to broiler farm operations (no history of previous exposure to broiler farm operations) and the farm site should be of elevated with good grip soil for buildings, free from water logging and flooding with reasonable wind flow and effective drain.
2. **Locality:** It should be located reasonably near to the market to procure the inputs and market the outputs, and away from other broiler farms and residential areas to avoid future problems.
3. **Accessibility:** Access to transport logistics (road access) for the smooth flow of input (chicks, feed and utilities) and output (live birds and manure).
4. **Water availability:** The land should have sufficient water sources and water should be free from all impurities to provide clean and safe drinking water to birds.
5. **Power supply:** The land should have access to electricity power to carry out the, brooding and machinery operations in a broiler farm.
6. **Labour availability:** Availability of cost effective labour is a desirable factor for site selection
7. **Approval:** The land should be an approved land for poultry farm operations. In area, where local rules and regulations exist for the same, necessary permission should be obtained from local authorities.

2. Financial Plan

Financial plan is nothing but, working out the budget requirement of establishing a broiler farm with the given specifications in the plan. The investment required to start a farm mainly composed of fixed investment. This investment has to be borne by the promoter or financial institution. Hence, a promoter or entrepreneur should understand the factors of fixed investment in detail and they are as follows,

1. Cost of land (own or lease)
2. Cost of land preparation (land levelling, water sources like bore well, water tank, electricity connection etc.)

3. Cost of construction of broiler house (on sq.ft basis)
4. Cost of equipment and other utilities
5. Cost of working capital (cost of chick, feed, utilities for first batch)

Considering all these factors, the entrepreneur should seek the help of a poultry consultant for detailed project report preparation for submitting to financial institutions.

Human Resource Planning

Intensive broiler farming is a scientific system of rearing, focusing the mass production, which also warrants considerable capital input. Because of that, the farm entrepreneur should consult a qualified poultry consultant before starting a farm business. The entrepreneur or the farm manager is also advised to undergo training on commercial broiler farming and acquaint him with the necessary basic facts about the production system to carry out the business on profitable basis.

Activity

1. A broiler farm's build up area requirements are as follows, and compute the total farm area requirement of the broiler farm with the construction co efficient of 0.35 and 0.40.
   a. Broiler houses : 3 Nos. (each measuring 7500 sq.ft)
   b. Mini feed mill : 500 sq.ft
   c. Labour quarters : 300 sq.ft
   d. Office : 200 sq.ft
2. A broiler farm's build up area requirements are as follows, and compute the total farm area requirement of the broiler farm with the construction co efficient of 0.25 and 0.30.
   a. Broiler houses : 4 Nos. (each measuring 10,000 sq.ft)
   b. Mini feed mill : 500 sq.ft
   c. Labour quarters : 300 sq.ft
   d. Feed store : 400 sq.ft
   e. Office : 200 sq.ft
3. Visit a contract broiler grower farm and an independent broiler farm, collect the data on their functional details and compare their production systems.

❏❏❏

Chapter 4

System of Rearing and Construction of Broiler Chicken Houses

Learning objectives:

1. *Discuss about the rearing systems of broilers and its merits and demerits*
2. *Design a open sided deep litter broiler house for tropical climatic conditions*

System of rearing of broilers

There are two systems of rearing practiced in broiler farming and they are :

Multiple - batch system

In this system, batches of day-old broiler chicks are purchased at regular intervals (weekly or bi-weekly) and reared up to market age. A characteristic feature of this system is at any point of time, birds of different ages in days or weeks are being reared in the same farm. Broiler farmers, who want to have a steady and continuous supply of broilers to the market at regular intervals, adopt this multiple-batch system, as it helps them to sell to the preferred retailers, and they need not depend on anybody to sell every batch of broilers produced. However, the major risk in this system of rearing is the rearing of different age groups of broilers in the same premises, leads to easy spread of infection, especially from adult to young birds. Presence of multiple batches increases the microbial load of the farm and affects the market age and weight, feed conversion efficiency, livability and overall production efficiency of the farm. Based on these limitations in the production efficiency, this system of rearing is almost obsolete in the Indian broiler production system.

All in – All out system

All in All out System is a scientific rearing method in which, one batch of day-old broiler chicks are received, reared up to optimum market age and weight in the farm and sold as one batch to the market, mostly to wholesalers. Then a time gap of two three weeks is provided to clean and disinfect the farm buildings and premises to rear the next batch. This period of gap is called as down time. Only one particular age group of broilers will be available in the farm, making it easier to rear, manage and control the spread of disease, as procedures to disinfect the premises can be applied promptly. However, a regular supply of broilers to the market at specified weekly intervals is not possible, and the producer or farmer has to depend mostly on wholesalers to sell his broilers by sacrificing his profit margin considerably. Considering this, the All-in-All-out system is preferred for large scale broiler production, compared to multiple batch system. All in All out system provides better efficiency of production and health management.

Broiler chicken houses

In broiler farming, farm building in the form of broiler houses constitutes nearly 50-60 per cent of the total capital expenditure depending on the type of house. The purpose of broiler housing is to protect the birds from extreme climate, theft, predatory animals, ensure comfortable rearing conditions, easy and better management to facilitate automation and to provide ideal microclimatic conditions for desirable performance.

In house optimal micro environmental conditions for rearing broilers

1	Temperature	22-25°C
2	Relative Humidity	40-60 percent
3	Ammonia	Less than 20 ppm
4	Deep Litter moisture	15-25 percent
5	Carbon di oxide	Less than 0.5 per cent
8	Distance between two broiler houses	60 feet

**Micro environment refers to the ambience within the broiler house*

Type of broiler houses

Considering the micro climatic requirements for broiler rearing, the broilers are reared in open sided deep litter houses; tunnel ventilated deep litter houses and environmentally controlled deep litter houses. However, considering the cost on construction and operation, farm size etc., open sided deep litter houses are highly recommended for Indian broiler farming systems.

Open sided deep litter house

Open sided means, the sides of long axis of the houses will be open, and closed only with chain link / mesh type material, allowing good cross ventilation. Since the sides are open, there will be limited control over microenvironments and it is critically influenced by macro environment prevails outside the house.

Deep litter is material spread over the floor of the house to provide cushioning effect to the broilers foot pad and it will also act as moisture absorbent material from broiler droppings. The commonly used litter materials are paddy husk and coir pith.

Floor space allowance

The floor space allowance for broiler depends on their market body weight, housing system and climatic conditions. Considering the open sided deep litter houses, the ideal floor space allowance is 0.5 sq.ft (450 sq.cm.) per kg live body weight. Considering the mean market weight of 2.0 to 2.20 kg of broiler, in Indian broiler farming conditions, 1 - 1.2 sq.ft per bird is the recommended floor space allowance. In summer, the space allowance may be increased by 10 percent and in winter, reduced by 10 percent by adjusting the number of birds in the available floor space. A broiler farm will be required a total floor space of 10,000 sq.ft and 12,000 sq.ft for 10,000 broiler batch size, at the rate of 1 and 1.2 sq.ft per bird floor space allowance.

Stocking density

Stocking density is defined as the quantity of live broilers (kg) is being reared per square metre area of floor space. It is a function of two factors, floor space allowance and market weight of bird and, expressed in kg per square metre. The ideal stocking density for open sided deep litter broiler houses will be 20 - 22 kg per square meter. However, in tunnel ventilated and environmentally controlled houses the stocking density recommendations are up to 30 - 32 kg per square meter.

Example :

A broiler farm's floor area is 10,000 sq.ft and the number of live broiler output of a batch, at the end of the market day is 9400 Nos. with the average live weight of 2.15 kg. Compute the stocking density of the batch.

1.	Total floor space available	:	10,000 sq.ft (10,000 /10.76 sq.ft = 930 sq.mt)
2.	Live broiler output	:	9400
3.	Mean market weight	:	2.15 kg
4.	Total live weight output	:	9400 x 2.15 kg = 20210 kg
5.	Stocking density	:	20210 / 930 = 21.73 kg per sq.mt.
6.	Realized floor space	:	10,000 / 9400 = 1.06 sq.ft per bird

Specifications for open sided deep litter broiler house

Orientation

The open sided deep litter broiler houses should be constructed with their *Long axis* in *East - West direction* to avoid direct sunlight falling into the building. However, ideal direction is, long axis should run parallel to the shadow of a vertical erected pole during the afternoon of the summer. This type of direction will not only prevent entry of sunlight in the animal shed, but also prevent the splashing of rainwater during monsoon.

Length and width

The ideal range of width for open sided deep litter house is 24-28 ft and width is always a limiting factor rather than length. Once the width is fixed, the length of the house is decided by the total floor space requirement and available dimension and topography of the land.

The reason for the wide range house width specifications is, that, width of the house will be decided based on the effective air movement prevails in the farm site. If air movement is high, width can be increased up to 28 feet. Otherwise in hot and humid areas it is desirable to reduce the width to 24 feet to facilitate effective cross ventilation.

The industrial broiler house length goes up to 300 - 350 feet based on the available length of the area. However, higher width will give the economic advantage in terms of cost per square foot of construction.

Floor

The floor of broiler houses should be raised one foot (30 cm) above the outer ground level to prevent seepage of water into the house. The floor should be made of cement for easy and efficient cleaning and disinfection process and to prevent damage by rodents and should be free from cracks and crevices. Improper flooring will leads to infection of micro-organisms, eggs of parasites, etc., which may cause outbreaks of disease.

Walls

The height of long axis side walls of open sided broiler houses should not be more than one foot (30 cm) above the floor level and the rest of area up to eave should be covered with wire mesh (1.25 x 1.25 cm, 20-22 gauge thick) or weld mesh (2.5 x 5.0 cm, 12-14 gauge thick) or chain link (2.5 cm, 12 gauge thick).

The width of the side wall should be 6 - 8 cm and the top of the sidewalls should be tapered and sloping inside (anti perch slope) to avoid perching of birds on the walls. The walls should be thoroughly cement-plastered to avoid cracks forming.

Doors

The doors of open sided houses should be 3 - 3.5 feet width and 6 ft height and for every 40-50 ft length one door should be provided with locking facilities from both sides. The door should be open inside the house for working ease.

Roof

In open sided broiler houses, the roof of may be thatched (coconut or palmyra leaves), Mangalore tiles, asbestos or new generation galvalume sheets. Thatched roofs are cheaper, eco friendly provide cool environment during hot season, but less durable and involves recurring expenditure after 3 years. Mangalore tile roofing is ideal for small and medium sized broiler houses and Galvalume sheet roofing for larger houses because of its cost and eco friendly advantages.

The height of the roof should preferably be 7-8 ft at eaves, and 11-12 ft at the ridge. The roof pitch should 4/12, it means 4 inch slope for 12 inches of run (run is half of the width). Thatched roofs may have a lower height of 6-7 ft at the eave and ridge to eave slope should be steeper for easy drain of rain water.

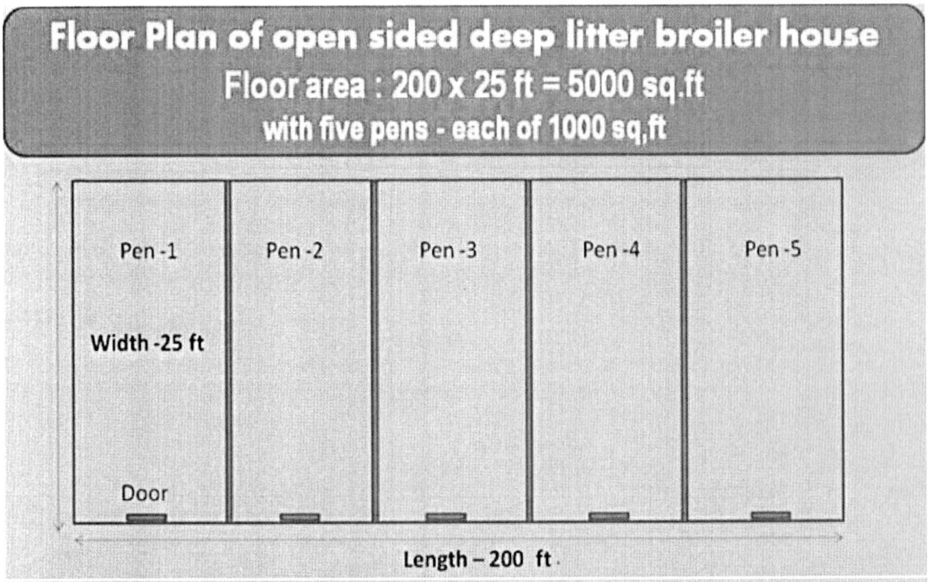

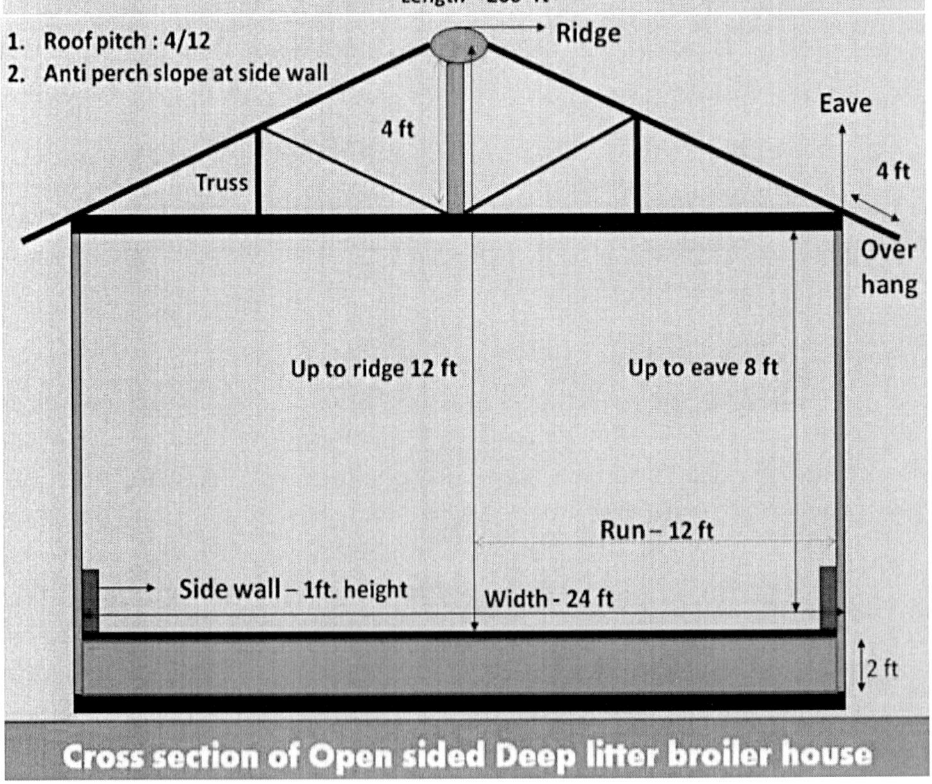

The extension of the roof at the eave is called as *Overhang* and should be at least 3-4 feet on either side to prevent direct sunlight and the splashing of rainwater into the buildings.

It is always beneficial to have the roof insulation to provide comfortable micro environment inside of the house. One of the simple and cost effective methods is painting white aluminium on roof to reflect the sun's rays and thereby reduce the heat build-up within the house. Insulation may be provided by a bed of straw on the top of the roof, or by having false roofing at the level of the eave.

Feeding and watering space allowance

Feeders and drinkers are devices used to keep the feed and water for the broilers to take feed and water. They may be conventional, semi-automatic or fully automatic. They can be linear or circular, and made of metal or plastic. Sufficient feeding and watering space per broiler has to be provided, depending on their age, feed and water intake and climatic conditions.

Feeder and water space allowances

Age of the broiler	Feeder space(cm)	Water space(cm)
0-2 weeks	3	1.5
3-4 weeks	5	2.5
Greater than 4 weeks	10	5.0

The feeder space available in a given feeder can be approximately calculated by multiplying the length by two for linear feeders or the diameter by three for circular feeders.

Commercially, feeders are available for chicks, growers and adult broilers in various volume capacities and they may be used according to the age of the broilers. Drinkers are also available in different sizes and volume capacities. They may be troughs or basins kept on the floor in the conventional manner, or hanging drinkers / fountain drinkers / nipple and cup drinker in an automatic system.

Watering space allowance should be increased by 20 percent during hot summer months. The drinkers and feeders should be uniformly distributed over the floor area so that the birds do not need to walk more than 150 cm. to reach a feeder or 200 cm. to a drinker. The height of the feeders and drinkers should be adjusted, so that the brim is at the same level of the back of the bird, to avoid wastage and spillage. For the same reason, they must be filled to only two-thirds of their capacity at any time.

However, it is worthy to mention that the birds lacks ability to swallow water by creating vacuum in side of the mouth, and swallowing the water by extending the neck high and through gravity. Consequently, water level in conventional floor drinkers (except nipple) are crucial. Water level below the half of the drinkers will not serve the purpose and it will put great amount of stress to the birds in their drinking process.

Broiler farm equipments

In planning a broiler farm, equipments accounts for 10-20 per cent of the capital expenditure depending on the system of housing, nature and quality of equipment. Level of automation, costing more to equipments but, it saves labour and provides convenience of management in long run.

Brooders

Brooder is set of arrangement used to provide warmth to young chicks during the first few weeks (2-3 weeks) of life. It consists of heating source in the form of light or heating coils, hovers (metal canopy - reflectors) to reflect the heat towards the chicks, chick guards, height adjustment devices for brooders and thermostats etc. The brooders can be classified as follows based on the heating source,

1. Electrical brooders
2. Gas brooders
3. Kerosene stove brooders
4. Coal pot brooders

Electrical brooder will be useful, where electricity is cheaper and heating source will be bulbs of Infra red or Incandescent or heating coils. Gas brooding and kerosene brooding can be adopted where electricity is costly and scarce.

In Indian broiler farming systems, cost effective coal pot brooders is being used. Fired and hot coal without any smoke is being put in to mud pot with two to three holes near neck being kept inside the broiler house to provide heat to the chicks. Number of pots will be decided by the area of house and number of chicks. One brooding arrangement will hold two mud pots to act as heating source to chicks.

Chick guards are the thin metal or hardboard or rigid plastic sheets or paper pulp mats with the height of 30 - 45 cm of varying length. They are arranged in a circular fashion to restrict the movement of chicks and to keep the chicks close to the heating source to avoid chilling. Circular arrangement of chick guards will avoid sharp corners and eliminate the chances of trampling of chicks during huddling.

Sprayer

Sprayer is one of the small but essential equipment in a broiler farm used to spray water, disinfectants and other cleaning solution inside and outside the broiler house.

Flame gun

Flame gun is equipment which will emit the fire flame to 2-3 ft long and it will be useful to destroy the dust, cob web, feathers and left over litter materials. It may be kerosene or gas operated. It will also be useful to clean the cages and crates and other metallic objects.

Crates

Crates are box like structures made of plastic or weld mesh used to transport the broiler to different houses and to the market and processing plant. Depending on the size it can hold 10-20 adult broilers and 50-100 young chicks. Use of plastic and collapsible crates will occupy less space and prevent the damage to the broilers during transport.

Weighing scales

Various range weighing scales and measuring jars are essential to weigh birds, feed, medicines and to measure disinfectant solutions etc., to do the precision in farming operations.

Foggers and sprinklers

Foggers are the equipments fitted inside the house to produce fog or mist like water spray, which will cool the broiler house. It needs

Broiler farm equipments

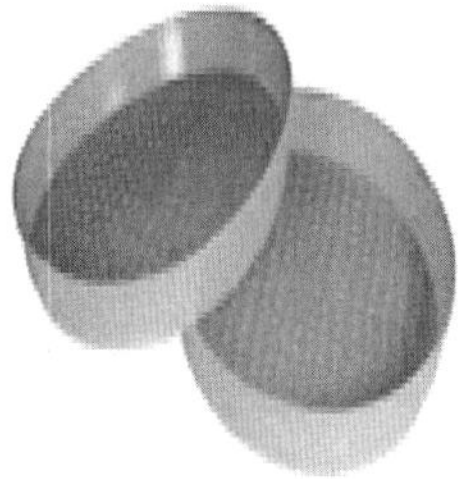

Chick feed tray

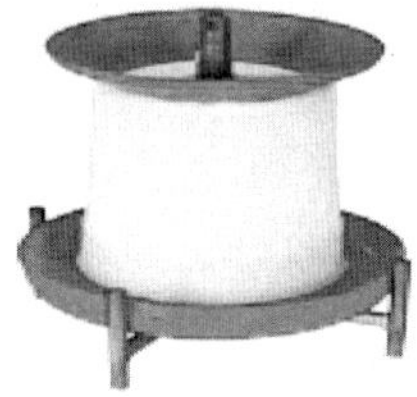

Chick Feeder - 2 kg capacity
20 Nos. for 1000 chicks

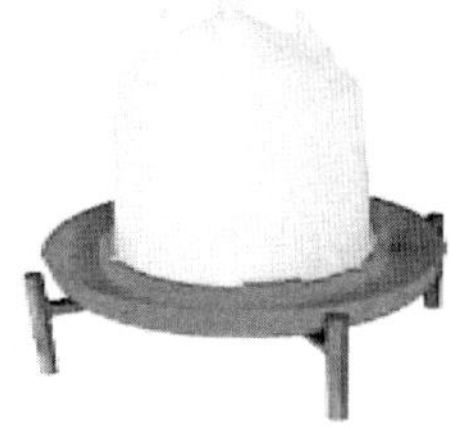

Chick drinker - 2.8 lit. capacity
20 Nos. for 1000 chicks

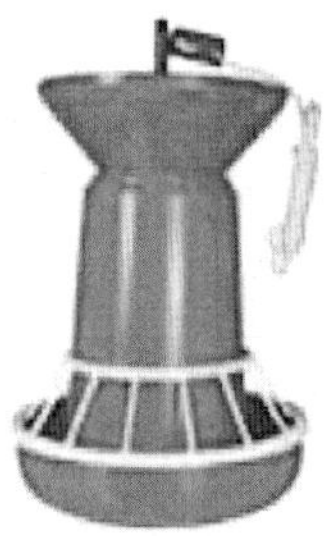

8 kg Capacity
25 Nos. for 1000 birds

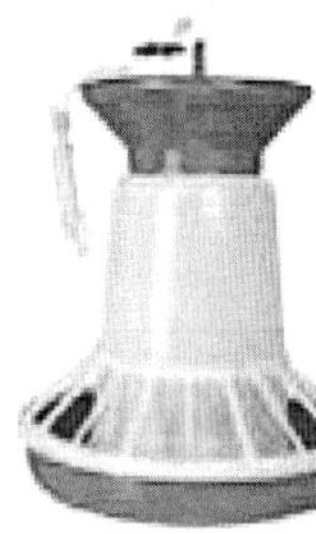

12 kg Capacity
18 Nos. for 1000 birds

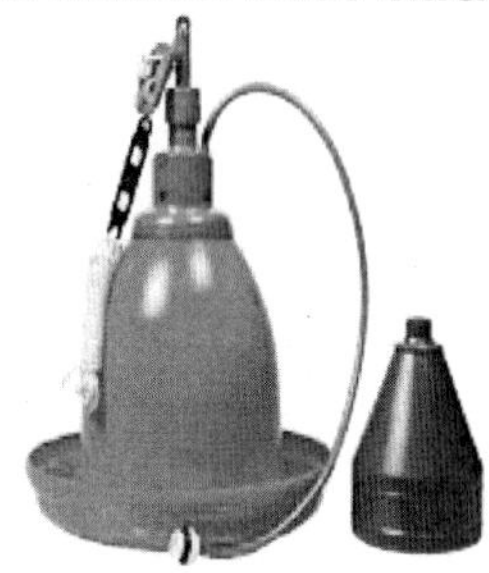

15- 20 Drinkers for 1000 birds

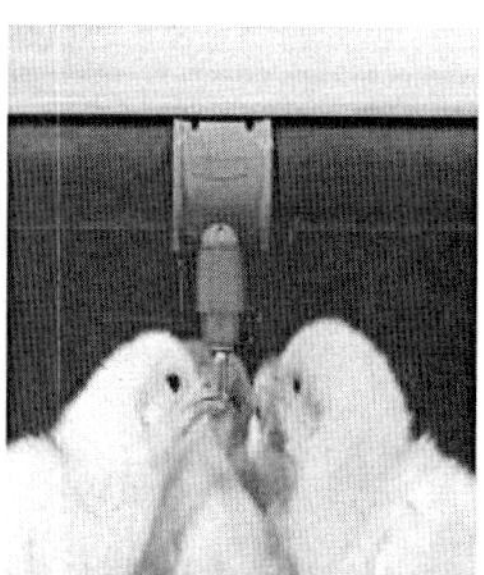

Nipple Drinkers

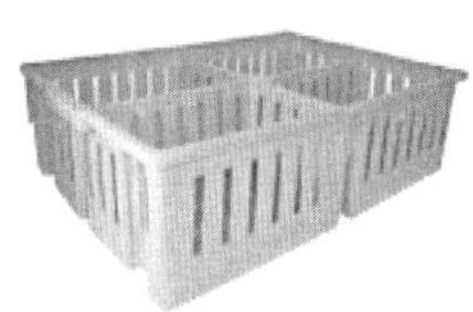

Chick box for DoC

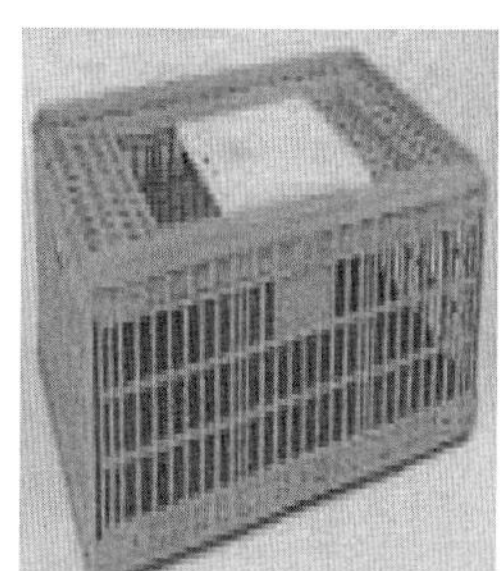

Broiler transport crates

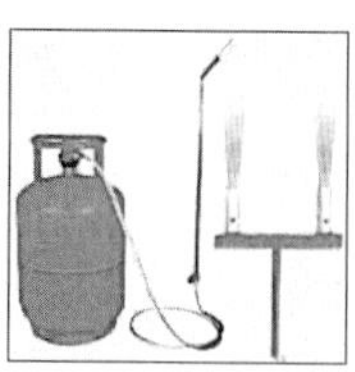

Flame Gun

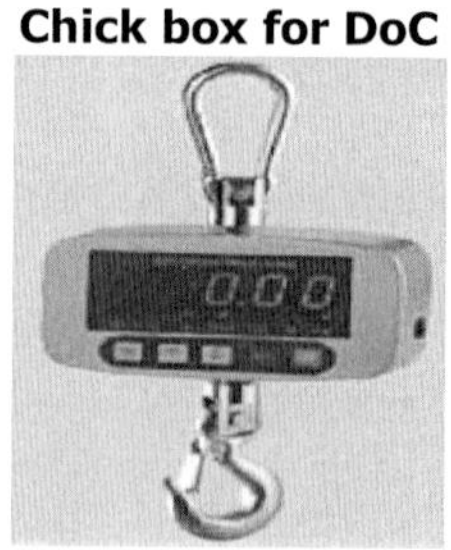

Weighing scale for broilers

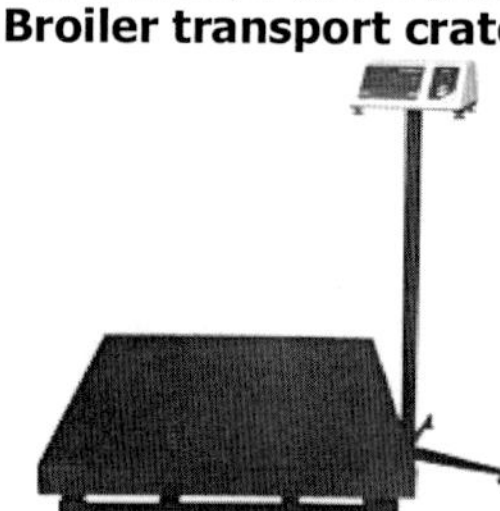

Weighing scale for feed

high pressure water pumps and filtered water and the functioning is intermittent based on outside environment temperature and relative humidity. Three to five minutes of fogging operation for every one hour is beneficial in hot and dry climatic conditions.

Sprinklers are fitted on the roof of the house (at ridge point) to sprinkle water on the roof, thereby it produces cooling effect inside the broiler house. It needs more water than foggers.

Vaccination and medication equipments

Vaccination and medication equipments include, syringes, needles, measuring glasses, ice flask and refrigerator or freezer to carry out proper vaccination and medication programme.

Activity

1. Design an open sided deep litter broiler house for 15,000 broilers batch size farm under all in all out system of rearing with suitable illustration for floor plan and cross sectional view.
2. Design a farm layout for 20,000 batch size broiler farm with two broiler houses, feed store, quarters and office under all in all out system of rearing.
3. Work out the stocking density and floor space allowance of batch of broilers in a commercial broiler farm with the following data

a. Total floor space	:	12,000 sq.ft
b. Day old Chick placement	:	10,000 Nos
c. Total live weight output at the end of 40 days	:	20245 kg
d. Livability	:	95 per cent

❏❏❏

Chapter 5

Brooding Management of Broiler Chicken

Learning objectives:

1. *List out the critical activities in brooding management of broiler chicken*
2. *Discuss the importance of brooding in broiler farm management*

Chick brooding

In natural outset, brooding is a common activity of care of chicks by the mother hen in their early stage. In commercial broiler farming, brooding is the art and science of rearing a large number of day old chicks, by providing enough warmth, feeding and watering arrangement in young age, usually, two to three weeks. The importance of brooding cannot be under estimated, because a newly hatched out chick does not have well developed thermoregulatory mechanism to maintain uniform body temperature (*homeostasis*). Therefore, it warrants artificial warmth, to get comfortable micro environment and to prevent death due to the chilling of body.

Broiler management is, sometimes called as *extended brooding management*, because, the rearing period of broiler chicken itself is six weeks. Considering the brooding period of 2-3 weeks, well brooding management covers nearly fifty per cent of rearing management of broilers.

Brooding period

In general, first two weeks of early life of chick is called as brooding period and sometimes it may extend up to third week, depending up on the climate of the area especially in winter. In extreme summer season, one week brooding will also serve the purpose.

Brooding methodology

Brooding is an integrated setup, consists of artificial heat sources and chick guards to keep the chicks near by the heat source, feeders and waters to feed the chicks on floor spread with litter material or in cages. The equipments required for brooding is as follows,

1. Brooder - Heat source (gas brooder/electrically operated brooder/ incandescent bulbs /infra red bulbs /hot coal pot etc.,).
2. Chick guard – It is 30-45 cm height, thin sheet, made of tin sheet, thick hard board, disposable paper pulp etc., to encircle the chicks in a confined area to provide the necessary warmthness to the chicks.
3. Chick feeder and drinkers - equipments used for feeding and watering the young chicks during brooding period (circular feeders /nipple /cup drinkers).
4. Litter material – Material used to spread on the floor to provide a cushioning effect to the foot pad of the chick and to absorb the moisture in the droppings.
5. Old news paper – To spread on the litter material to prevent the eating of litter material by young chicks.

Preparation of brooding setup

Generally, preparation of brooding starts two days before the arrival of chicks. Careful arrangement of brooding involves following steps.

1. Complete cleaning, washing and disinfection of broiler house, three weeks before the arrival of chicks and keep the sheds empty for at least two weeks.
2. Identify the brooding areas and it may be a part of shed (partial house brooding) or one corner of the shed (corner house brooding), which is depending on the need, convenience and brood size.
3. Decide the size of brood and brood size should not exceed 400 chicks per brooding setup.
4. Comfortable brooder floor space requirement is 250 sq.cm per chick for two weeks during brooding period.
5. For example, circular chick guard with 12 feet width diameter will offer optimum floor space for 400 chicks.

6. Based on the size of the brood (number of chicks in a brood) arrange the chick guard in a circular fashion and brooder heat source in the centre of the brooder area.
7. Diameter of the circular brooder setup will decide the floor space available in the brooder setup and it can be calculated by using the formulae for area of circle (pi r^2, pi = 3.14, r = radius of the circle).
8. Spread of litter in the brooding area, one or two days before the arrival of chicks and spread of old and clean news paper.
9. Keep the height of brooders and hovers one foot from floor on first day and slowly increase the height and it can be removed at the end of two weeks based on the room temperature.
10. The cleaned and sanitized feeders and drinkers should be placed in brooders and they have to be arranged alternatively in a "cart wheel spokes" like fashion for easy availability of feed and water to chicks.
11. The number of feeder and drinkers should be based on the number of chicks and at the rate of one feeder and drinker for 40-50 chicks.
12. Chicks, feed may also be offered feed in chick feed trays/chick box lids/egg filler flats to encourage feeding.

Receiving of Day old chicks

In general, day old chicks will be dispatched from the hatchery at the evening and it will reach the farm at early morning to provide comfort during transport. As soon as the chicks are arrived in the farm, the baby chicks should be immediately transfer from chick box and placed under brooder on count basis and discard the chick box.

Two hours before of arriving of the chicks, heating source should be *on* in brooder and water should be filled in drinkers and do not fill up the feeders. The ideal first day brooding temperature is 95 $^{\circ}$ F and it should be reduced 1° F per day and 7th and 14th day it should be at 88 and 81° F. The thumb rule for using incandescent bulbs is providing 1 watt per chick. It is always advisable to check the temperature at the brooder setup for maximum comfort.

Once the baby chicks started drinking water, after an hour, feed shall be sprinkled in feeder trays and news paper spread, to encourage the chicks to take feed. After that, regular feeders should be filled with feed. Here it is important to mention that for the first two weeks chicks should be given cooled boiled water with 10 gram of glucose with 1 g of electrolyte per litre of water as additives.

Quality of brooding

Quality of brooding is assessed by the chick movement pattern within the brooder, feed intake of chicks, uniformity in growth and livability of chicks. Pattern of movements of chicks under brooder is the right indicator of the well being of the chicks. The chicks should be active, move freely, scratch, take the feed and water and make chirping noise.

If the chick distribution under the brooder is not uniform, correct the brooder temperature and ventilation accordingly. It is necessary to verify whether the warmth given is sufficient for the chicks.

A thermometer kept at the level of the birds will indicate the air temperature. However, a more practical way of assessing the adequacy of the warmth is by watching the behaviour and distribution of the chicks within the chick guard arrangement. If they crowd under or near the source of heat, the warmth is not sufficient. Then, additional heat may be added to the hover, or the height of the hover may be reduced. If chicks have moved to the periphery and are reluctant to come under the heat source, the temperature is too high. Then the hover must be pushed up or a bulb shall be removed. If the chicks feel comfortable at the given temperature, they walk actively throughout the area and some will rest with their head on one side posture called "chick comfort". In practice, the heat source should be put on for 23½ hours in a day for the first 3 days, and switched off for only 30 minutes during night for adapting the chicks to dark. Later on, heat may be given during the night only, up to the end of the second or third week, depending on the season. It may be restricted to one week only during peak summer and extended to three weeks during winter or rainy seasons. In winter and rainy seasons, it is advisable to close the sides of the house with thick curtains.

Assessment of the feed intake of chicks

To assess the feed consumption of chicks is highly essential to ensure the uniformity in weight gains in broiler chicken. *Crop fill* test is an easy test assess the feed consumption of young chicks. Collect 30 chicks randomly in a brood, and check the crop for its emptiness or fullness. Full and soft crop indicates the intake of feed and water and full and hard indicates the intake of feed and lack of water intake. The target for crop fill test is 100 per cent within 48 hours of brooding.

Growing of broilers is a continuous process after brooding of broiler chicks. From the brooding set up, newspaper spread on the litter may be removed after 3-4 days and the chick guard arrangement may be dismantled at the end of brooding period. During brooding, clean, potable water should be provided. In the early morning, the first duty in the daily routine is, the drinkers should be emptied, cleaned and filled with fresh water. Water must be given twice daily and feed four times a day. Fill the feeders only to two-thirds of their capacity to avoid feed wastage. Water spill over litter should be avoided. If conventional chicken drinkers and plastic basins are used, have one spare set and clean and dry the used set in the sun every day.

Brooding arrangement in a commercial broiler farm

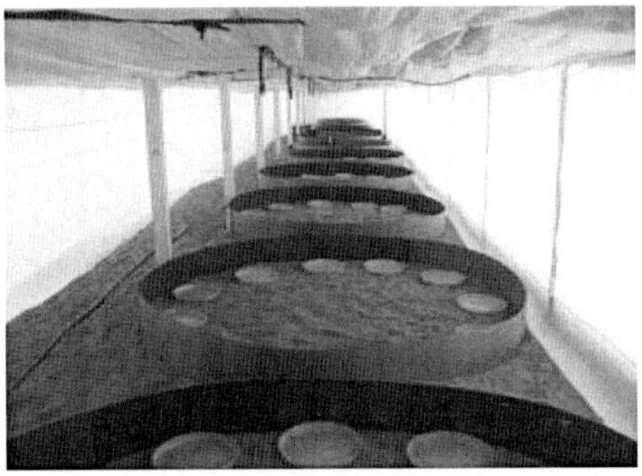

Partial house brooding

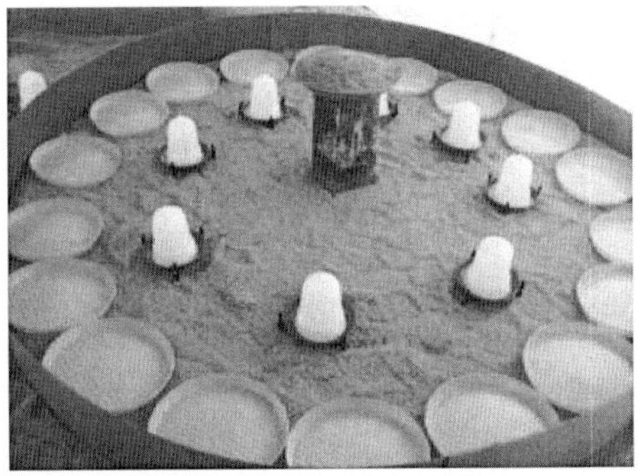

Arrangement of brooder

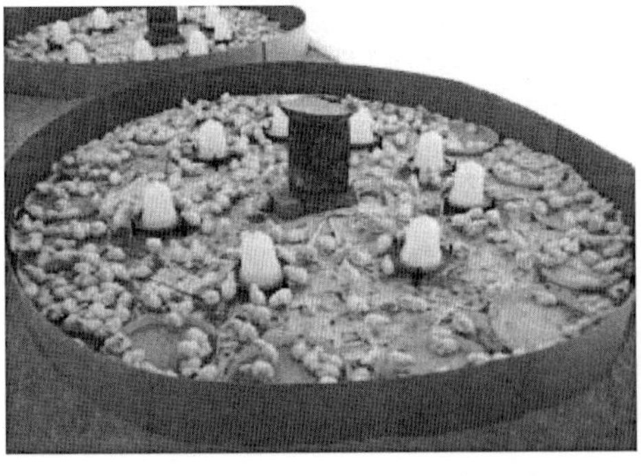

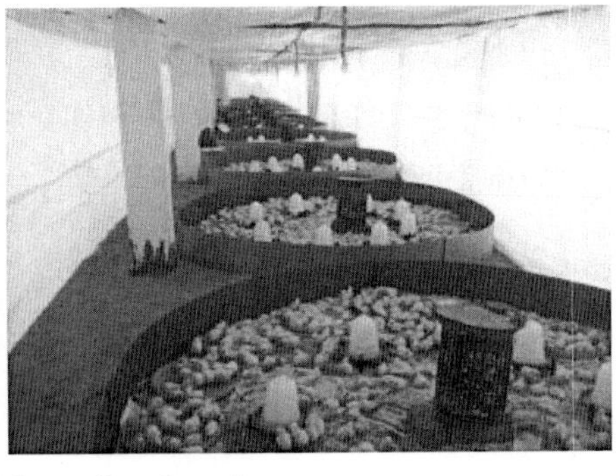

Individual and row of brooding in a farm

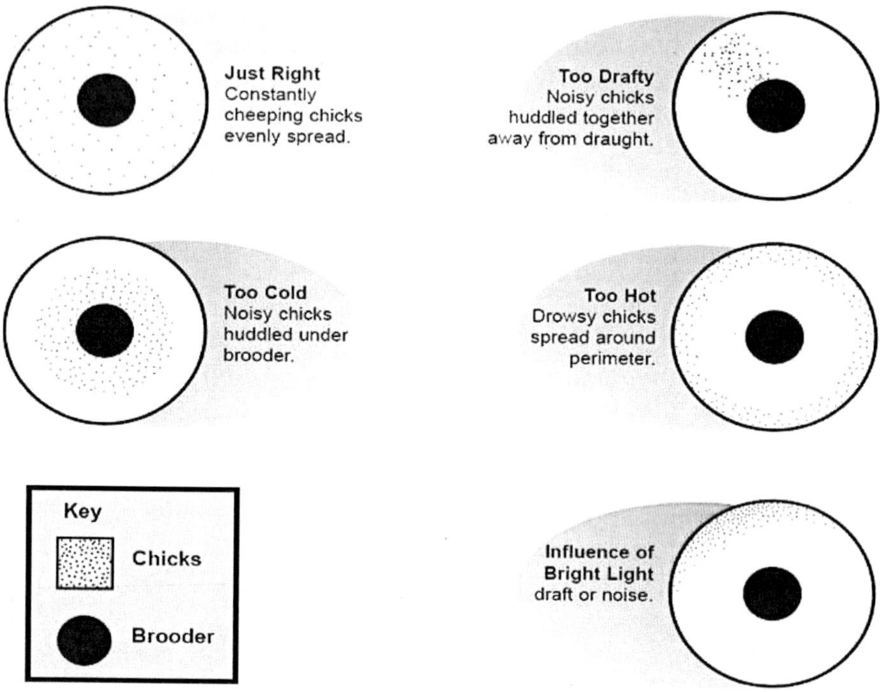

Pattern of chick movement in brooding

Source : Cobb - Broiler managment guide

Activity

1. Arrange a brooder setup for 5000 broiler chick placement with suitable illustrations and calculate the following,
   a) Number of brooding arrangements
   b) Chicks per brooder set up
   c) Area of a single brooder setup
   d) Floor space allowance per chick
   e) Number of feeders and waters required.

Chapter 6

Feeding and Rearing Management of Broiler Chicken

Learning objectives:

1. *List out the critical steps in feeding management of broilers*
2. *Discuss the various broiler feed specifications*
3. *Discuss the importance of rearing management in broiler chicken farming*

Feed is the most crucial input in intensive broiler farming system and it is the single largest cost item in total cost of production of broiler meat. In any industrial broiler farming system, feed accounts for 70-75 per cent of the total cost of production. Quality and cost of feed affects the production performance and thereby cost of production. Escalation of feed prices (cost of feed ingredients) is alarming in recent past, creating lot of research focus on preparing cost effective (*least cost*), quality feed, by optimizing the feed formulae, there by maximize or optimize the production efficiency. In large and integrated broiler farm operations, feed is being prepared in their own facility in an attempt to reduce the feed cost with quality assurance. An entrepreneur, who wants to be successful in his broiler venture, should understand the basics of broiler feeding in terms of

1. Nutrients requirement of broiler chicken: It depends on chiefly, the type of bird (broiler), age of the bird like, pre starter feed (0-2 weeks), starter feed (3-4 weeks) and finisher feed (5-6 weeks), climatic profile of the area (tropical or temperate) and bird's performance.
2. Feed ingredients: In industrial broiler farming, feed ingredients are more or less uniform throughout production areas; choices are inevitable considering the availability, quality and cost factors, in which selection and quality control of feed ingredients is a critical process in feed preparation.

3. Feed formulation: Feed formulation is a scientific process which, needs understanding about the requirement and nutrient profile of the feed ingredient and formulator should know to how best to meet out the requirements by mixing various feed ingredients and at the same time minimize the feed cost without compromising the quality and production performance.
4. Feed Milling: Feed milling is the actual feed preparation process in feed mills, here the challenge is to prepare a feed, may be mash / pellet / crumbles without affecting the quality of feed ingredients (nutrient quality/wastage).
5. Feeding of broilers: It is the final step in feeding management, in which to how to feed broilers without wasting the finished feed is the challenge.

In all these steps, there is great scope for application for Good Husbandry Practices, following a structured programme of GHP in feeding management will result in improved performance and least cost of feed per unit of meat output.

Broiler feeding standards

The broiler feeding standards prescribes the nutrient requirement of broiler chicken during various stages of age and growth to maximize/ optimize the performance in cost effective way. Recommendations of Bureau of Indian Standards (BIS) shall be taken as a model for that purpose. The slight modifications can be made based on the commercial strain performance and the climate of the area in question.

Bureau of Indian Standards (1992) - Broiler chicken feed

S.No.	Nutrient	Broiler type	
		Starter (0-3 wks)	Finisher (4-6 wks)
1	Crude protein (%), Min.	23	20
2	M.E. (Kcal/kg), Min.	2900	3000
3	Crude fibre (%) Max.	6	6
4	Calcium (%) Min.	1.2	1.2
5	Available phosphorus (%) Min.	0.50	0.50
6	Lysine (%) Min.	1.20	1.00
7	Methionine (%), Min.	0.50	0.35
8	Linoleic acid (%) Min.	1.00	1.00
9	Sodium chloride (%) Max.	0.60	0.60

However, considering the rate of growth of broilers in various stages, commercially, phase feeding at three levels are practiced in tropical broiler industry and the recommendations of the same is as follows :

Critical nutrient requirement of broilers in tropics

Nutrient	Type of broiler feeds		
	Pre -Starter 0-10 days	**Starter 11-25 days**	**Finisher 26 days to market**
Metabolizable energy (Kcal ME/kg diet)	3000	3100	3200
Crude protein (%) Min.	23	21	19
Lysine (%) Min.	1.40	1.20	1.10
Methionine (%) Min.	0.62	0.52	0.49
Threonine (%) Min.	0.89	0.83	0.77
Tryptophan (%) Min.	0.22	0.20	0.18
Calcium (%) Min.	1.0	1.0	1.0
Available phosphorous (%) Min.	0.50	0.46	0.42
Sodium chloride (%) Min.	0.50	0.50	0.50
Linoleic acid (%) Min.	1.2	1.20	1.2
Fibre (%) Max.	6.0	6.0	6.0

Common broiler feed ingredients

Though, there are number of conventional and unconventional feed ingredients are used in poultry feed, in industrial broiler farming, commonly used broiler feed ingredients and their inclusion levels are summarized below.

Inclusion levels and Nutrient composition of common poultry feed ingredients

Name of the ingredients	Inclusion levels	C. P. (%)	M.E. (Kcal/ kg)	C.F. (%)	Ca (%)	NPP (%)	Lysine (%)	Methionine (%)
Maize (Corn)	60	8.9	3300	2.3	0.03	0.1	0.22	0.18
Jowar	30	10.3	3256	2.4	0.05	0.011	0.21	0.16
Bajra	30	11.6	2850	4	0.05	0.12	0.24	0.16
Wheat	30	11.0	3120	3	0.05	0.1	0.33	0.18
Broken rice	40	8.5	2900	3	0.08	0.1	0.21	0.14
Rice bran	30	12.9	2400	12	0.05	0.22	0.39	0.13
Deoiled rice bran (DORB)	40	13.5	1900	14	0.07	1.01	0.62	0.28
Vegetable (Rice Bran) oil	06	-	7800	-	-	-	-	-
Soybean meal (SE)	40	42.0	2420	6.5	0.29	0.26	2.59	0.52
Groundnut meal (SE)	30	43.0	2100	12.2	0.17	0.18	1.61	0.44
Sunflower meal (SE)	30	27.0	1900	24.9	0.37	0.91	1.14	0.65
Fish Meal (45%)	10	45.0	2460	1	5.39	2.99	2.27	0.87
Meat meal - 50%	04	50.0	2200	2	6.27	3.1	2.61	0.69
Di-calcium phosphate	03	-	-	-	22	18	-	-
Calcite	03	-	-	-	36	-	-	-
Shell grit / lime stone	03	-	-	-	36	-	-	-

SE- Solvent Extracted

Feed formulation

Generally, broiler feed formulation is done by nutritionist, specialized in poultry science by using principle of least cost feed formulation with the use of computer. To prepare a balanced , least cost, and quality feed, one should have thorough understanding about the nutrient requirement of broilers, nutrient composition and inclusion level of various feed ingredients, and cost factors of feed ingredients. Basically, the broiler feed consists of 50-60 per cent grains as energy source, 25-35 per cent oil meals, fish and meat meal as protein source and 1-3 per cent mineral sources. Additives will be added as per the requirement. The broiler farm entrepreneur should always consult a poultry consultant for issues regarding feed formulation and preparation for better results.

Model broiler feed formulations for tropical countries

Feed ingredient	Pre Starter		Starter		Finisher	
	1	2	1	2	1	2
Maize	20	30	20	30	20	35
Jowar	10	10	10	-	10	10
Millets	10	-	10	10	10	-
Broken Rice	15.8	14.5	18	17	20	14
Fat / Oil	-	2	0.8	3.5	1.7	5.5
Full Fat Soya	10	-	16	-	20	-
Soyabean meal	25	40	16	36	9	32
Dry unsalted fish	5	-	5	-	5	-
Meat cum bone meal	2.5	-	2.5	-	2.5	-
Calcite	1.2	1.7	1.2	1.8	1.3	1.9
Di calcium phosphate	0.5	1.8	0.5	1.7	0.5	1.6
Total (kg)	**100**	**100**	**100**	**100**	**100**	**100**

Addition of molasses will improve the palatability, flavor of the feed, reduce the dustiness and improves the pellet quality. Molasses and oil incorporation in the feed offers beneficial effect during summer. Addition of oil / fat will the increase the energy level of feed will provide cooling effect due to higher metabolic water yield, increased energy concentration will reduce the feed intake and improves the feed efficiency. Marginal deficit of lysine and methionine can meet out by addition of synthetic preparations. In practical feed formulations, if the levels of protein, energy, lysine and methionine are achieved, there is no need to check other nutrients and mostly deficit will not occur in other nutrients, even if is so it can be met adding synthetic feed additives.

Broiler feed milling

Broiler feed milling is mostly an engineering process, which needs full fledge feed mills. It consists of batch weighing scales, grinders, mixers and quality control lab. Broiler integrators operate their feed mill with experienced feed mill experts and poultry consultants for better results. Feed cost shall be reduced considerably in own feed preparation; however the farmers should be financially capable of bearing the feed ingredients inventory. When feed ingredients are available locally, own feed preparation will be profitable.

Broiler integrators are capable of investing more on ingredient procurement, feed preparation and milling operations because of their volume, will reap substantial reduction in the cost of feed. They can make use of high tech milling operations, resulting in quality assurance. Broiler feed shall be prepared in three forms namely crumbles, pellets and mash. Commercial broiler farming industry mostly using crumbles (pre starter feed) and pellets for its superiority in quality.

Feeding of broilers

Broiler is a fast growing bird and efficient energy converter. Feeding of broilers should be done *ad libitum* basis (free choice or no restriction over feed intake) in three phases. During the first two weeks of age, broiler pre starter feed may be offered, followed by starter feed for 3 - 4 weeks and, finisher feed from five weeks to market age. During feeding and watering, the birds should not be disturbed much. If possible, the same person should attend to each batch. Feeding and watering may also be done at the same time every day to minimize stress. Take all possible steps to avoid feed wastage. During growing phase, grower and adult feeders and drinkers have to be used specifically. Provide an adequate number of feeders; make provisions to adjust the height of feeders so that the brim of the feeder or drinker is at the same level as the back of the growing broiler. Watch the growth of the broilers up to market age by weighing random samples at the end of every week to make sure that they are gaining weight normally, and that there is no sudden drop in growth rate. If the growth rate is lower than normal, check the quality of the feed for the presence of toxins, adequacy of protein and critical amino acid levels. The possibility of any sub-clinical infection should also be monitored. Watch the daily consumption of feed and water, as any drastic change has to be investigated.

Based on the above table, it is evident that the cumulative over all feed conversion efficiency and body weight of commercial broiler at sixth week are 1.74 and 2.355 kg. The body weight, feed intake, feed efficiency will vary slightly with commercial strains. The entrepreneur should take the standards in the management guides for the specific strain in use.

Body weight, weight gain and feed consumption of commercial broilers

Generalized performance of a commercial broiler

Age (week)	Body weight (g)	Weight Gain (g)		Feed consumption (g)		Feed Conversion		Avg. daily feed intake (g)	Avg. daily gain (g)
		Weekly	Cumu-lative	Weekly	Cumu-lative	Weekly	Cumu-lative		
1	175	135	135	149	149	1.10	1.10	21.3	19.29
2	440	265	400	322	471	1.22	1.18	46.0	37.86
3	795	355	755	515	986	1.45	1.31	73.6	50.71
4	1250	455	1210	764	1750	1.68	1.45	109.1	65.00
5	1770	520	1730	1011	2761	1.94	1.60	144.4	74.29
6	2355	585	2315	1313	4074	2.24	1.76	187.6	83.57

Hatch weight: 40 gram

Water and feed consumption will vary depending on the season. Feed consumption will decrease and water consumption will increase during summer, and during winter or the rainy season, water consumption will decrease and feed consumption will go up, due the increased maintenance energy requirements. Since birds eats for their energy requirements, energy content of the feed will also have substantial influence on feed intake and feed conversion efficiency. Accordingly, feed efficiency will be better during summer and poorer during winter.

Water management of broilers

Watering management of broilers is the most neglected area by most of commercial farmers. They are not considering the water as critical nutrient. Since the metabolic activity of broiler is high, due to its high growth performance, the intake of water will also be high. In general, broiler will take twice the quantity of feed as water intake. For example, when the feed intake per day is 150 gram, the water intake will be 300 ml per bird per day, when the temperature will be around 28-32 °C. When the temperature increases above 35°C, water intake will be of three fold of feed intake. Considering that, good quality water should always available for broiler chicken at all times with adequate drinkers in number and volume.

Mean feed and water intake of broiler chicken

Age(week)	Feed consumption per day (g)	Water consumption per day (ml)
1	21	40
2	46	60
3	73	140
4	109	210
5	144	300
6	187	370

Guidelines for water quality management in broiler farming

1. Water quality management starts from the farm site selection and before selecting a site, water quality of the site is to be tested for its physical, chemical and microbiological quality.
2. Medium to deep bore well water is highly suitable for broiler farming, because of its consistency in quality, irrespective of change of water table during summer and rainy seasons.

3. Farm size is the deciding factor for total water quantity requirement. When calculating the drinking water requirement of farm, take the standards of one litre of water per bird per day. (example: 10,000 batch size broiler farm requires 10,000 litres water storage tanks, considering the buffer water storage capacity)
4. Use of water sanitizers is recommended, when ever water quality is being affected.

Critical water quality standards for broiler farm

S.No.	Quality parameters	Maximum Acceptable level
1	pH	6.5-7.5
2	Total Dissolved Solids (TDS)	Less than 1000
3	Total Hardness	110 ppm
4	Calcium	60 mg per litre
5	Chloride	250 mg per litre
6	Sodium	50 mg per litre
7	Nitrate	25 mg per litre
8	Total bacterial count	100 CFU per ml
9	Coliform count	50 CFU per ml

Source: National Research Council, 1994

Litter management

In Indian broiler farming systems, since the broilers are rearing in deep litter system, effective litter management is highly essential for overall performance.

Functions of litter material in broiler rearing

1. To provide a cushioning effect to the foot pad of broiler chicken
2. To absorb moisture in broiler excreta
3. To provide an insulation from cold floor temperatures.

Qualities of a good litter material

1. It must be cheap and locally available
2. It must absorb moisture from droppings quickly

3. It must release moisture and dry up quickly
4. It must have least tendency to form cakes
5. It must be non toxic and free from mould growth

The commonly used materials as litter are paddy husks, coir pith, groundnut hulls, sawdust, wood-shavings, chopped straw and sugar cane bagasse. The choice of litter material depends mostly on cost and local availability of the material.

The ideal initial height of litter spread is 5 cm during summer and 7 cm in winter. The litter should be kept as dry as possible by avoiding water spillage from drinkers and close the curtains during windy rains. Caked and wet litter material should be removed quickly. Before adding fresh litter, remove the caked litter and rack the litter with litter racker and allow it to dry.

Litter moisture is a very good indicator of litter quality. The ideal litter moisture level is 20-25 per cent. To assess moisture levels in the litter, squeeze a handful. If the litter forms a cake, the moisture level is too high. If it crumbles into fine dust, the moisture level is very low, which will make the environment dusty. When the moisture level is optimum, it remains as a loose mass.

The major problems due to excess moisture in litter are

1. More ammonia and respiratory problems
2. Incidence of coccidiosis
3. Breast blisters, dermatitis and foot pad problems
4. Contamination of feed and water

There are number of factors affecting the litter quality and during the time of trouble shooting, those factors should be monitored

1. Over crowding
2. Lack of ventilation
3. Leaky drinkers and splashing of rain water
4. Excess fibre in feed and wet litter problems

Recycling of litter

Recycling of litter is practiced in some places due to cost and scarce of litter. Heaping and reheaping is the method used for recycling and heat generated in the heaping of litter will inactivate the microbes present in the litter and make it safe. However, recycled litter is always inferior to fresh litter and use of recycled litter shall be avoided for hygienic broiler farming operations.

Lighting for broilers

To provide warmth for brooding, artificial lighting has to be given up to three weeks in brooding. Afterwards, it is recommended to provide a total photo-period of 16 hours per day (a photo-period is natural daylight + artificial lighting from roof level - one 60 w bulb for every 10 square metre area). Lighting beyond the natural day length for a certain period is recommended to facilitate additional feed intake and improved growth rate. As birds have the habit of compensating feed intake, lighting beyond 16 hours per day will not be beneficial and will only increase the electricity cost. However, during summer, continuous night lighting except for a one-hour break is recommended to allow the birds to take feed in night.

Summer management of broiler chicken

In Indian climatic conditions, it is common to have high ambient temperature (inland - hot and dry) and in some areas often accompanied with high humidity (coastal - hot and humid). In these situations, acute heat stress will substantially affect the overall productivity of a broiler flock. At environmental temperatures above 35°C (95°F) heat stress induced mortality and marked production losses are common, however, at lesser temperatures; heat stress is often viewed as a predisposing cause for chronic losses in growth of broilers. Clear understanding of heat stress and managemental strategies to overcome the heat stress is highly essential for tropical broiler production systems.

Physiology of thermo regulation in broilers

Chicken is homoeothermic in nature, and they try to maintain a relatively constant deep body temperature (41-42°C) irrespective of environmental temperature. The thermo neutral zone or "zone of comfort" is a particular range of environmental temperature, in which, birds do not change their behaviour or show signs of discomfort and use minimum amount of metabolic energy to maintain homoeothermic range of body temperature.

In thermo neutral zone, body temperature is maintained by the thermal equation (heat production=heat loss). Increasing environmental temperature causes hyperthermia. Action on reducing hyperthermia can be activated by increasing heat dissipation and or decreasing heat production. Chicken, unlike most other animals, do not have sweat glands to aid in heat loss. The chicken removes excess body heat in four ways through the signals of thermoregulatory centre located at hypothalamus. Body heat can be lost by *radiation* from the skin surface through the air to another object. Heat can be directly transferred by *conduction* to cooler objects with which the bird is in contact, such as litter. Body heat is also lost to the surrounding air by *convection*. When the environmental temperatures are between 30 - 35°C (86°F and 95°F), radiation, conduction, and convection heat losses are usually adequate to maintain the bird's body temperature. In these temperature zones, the bird dilates the blood vessels of the skin, wattles, and comb to bring the internal body heat to the skin surface to facilitate conductive, convective, and radiative heat loss. Birds at floor will search for cool places in the house, spreads the litter and squats to increase the conductive and convective heat loss by increasing the body surface area.

When environmental temperature approaches the body temperature of the bird, 41°C (106°F), the efficiency of these heat loss mechanism diminish. At this point the *evaporation of water* from the respiratory tract and mouth becomes the major heat loss mechanism of the bird. Birds will begin to pant (open mouth breathing), or hyperventilate to increase evaporative cooling. When panting fails to prevent the rise in body temperature, the bird becomes listless, comatose, followed by death due to heat stroke. Birds raised from young age at high environmental temperatures will acclimatize to higher environmental temperature variations and extremes and can maintain good productivity even in high ambient temperatures to a certain extent. The non-acclimatized flock exposed to rapid increase in environmental temperature (acute heat stress) has the greatest loss in production and mortality.

Effects of heat stress

One of the primary effects of high environmental temperature on a flock is reduced feed intake. Reduction in appetite is the birds' effort to reduce energy intake in response to the increase in environmental temperature by neuro signals from hypothalamus and thyroid (T_3- Triiodothyronine- suppression of hunger centre), thereby reducing the energy obtained from feed. Birds may use body fat as a source of energy that produces less heat increment than digestion/metabolism of proteins or carbohydrates in the feed. The reduced feed intake and subsequent deficit of other critical nutrients quickly affect the productivity of the flock. Growth retardation occurs in growth of broilers. The nasal passages function is to filter dust and bacteria from air entering the respiratory tract, and this system is by-passed when birds resort to open-mouth breathing (panting). This can lead to an increased incidence of secondary bacterial respiratory infections. Factors influencing the extent of production losses from heat stress are:

1. The maximum temperature to which the flock was exposed,
2. Duration of the high temperatures,
3. The rate of temperature change
4. Relative humidity of the air.

Problems of open sided houses

1. Extreme hot and cold are problems in summer and winter
2. Humidity - Coastal, rainy season will have above 70 per cent relative humidity and inland and summer may have less than 40 per cent
3. High mean day time temperature (35-42°C) and severe fluctuation of temperature
4. Seasonality of air velocity
5. Inefficiency of mechanical ventilation

Key points of housing design in open sided houses

- Orient the long axis of poultry house in an east-west direction to minimize solar heating and direct access to sunlight

- In open sided houses, width of house will be a limiting factor, so keep the optimum width (24-28 ft) based on , temperature, humidity, wind velocity, type of house and nature of bird for effective cross ventilation
- Increased air movement over the birds by cooler fans / exhaust to produce a *wind chill* effect, which will cool birds even without a drop in the house temperature.
- Roof overhangs should be sufficient (3-5 ft) to protect the birds from strong sunrays.
- Poultry houses in tropics should have good roof insulation, (If possible with "false roof" to reduce the conduction of heat) with the support of foggers and cooler systems.
- Grow grass with sprinklers around the house to cool incoming air and reduce the reflection of heat into open houses. Bare ground can reflect a large amount of heat into the house.
- Place water sprinklers on the roof ridge to remove heat from the roof.
- Drinking water stored in overhead water tanks can get very hot. These tanks should be painted with white colour, so as to reflect the solar radiation and avoid direct sunlight.
- Remove any unwanted large metal objects around the houses (machinery, vehicles, and nest boxes) which could radiate heat into open houses.

Nutritional management of the heat stressed flock

Heat-stressed flocks usually experience a loss in appetite. This reduced feed intake can be compensated by formulating a nutrient rich feed. The actual energy requirement of the bird is reduced at high environmental temperatures because the birds do not require energy to maintain its body temperature, but all the other dietary nutrients (i.e., protein, minerals, and vitamins) remain the same. The following feeding regimen is generally considered as appropriate during periods of stress due to increased temperature. The commercial broiler farmer should anticipate weather changes through regular forecasting system to make necessary corrections in the management schedule,

- The by-product of the digestion/metabolism of feed is the production of body heat (Heat increment/Specific Dynamic

Action). It is a recognized fact that fat has the lowest heat increment, when compared to proteins and carbohydrates, the heat load of the bird can be reduced by including dietary fat up 3-5 percent and it will also offer more metabolic water which will have a cooling effect during the summer stress and fat added feed is more palatable.

- Ensure that the non-energy nutrients, such as amino acids, vitamins, and minerals are increased in the formula in proportion to the decrease in feed intake.
- When the nutrient density of the formula is increased to compensate for the reduction of feed intake, the protein content of the feed may be reduced by about 0.5 percent than the standard. At the same time intake of the essential and critical amino acids (lysine, methionine and threonine) can be optimized by providing enough quantities of synthetic amino acid preparations.
- Avoid feeding of birds about three hours before ambient temperature is expected to exceed 36°C (99°F). Adjust the lighting schedule to encourage the feed consumption in the night and early morning. Midnight feeding or an intermittent lighting program can encourage feed consumption at night.
- Inclusion of Vitamin A 12,000 IU and Vitamin E -150 mg per kg diet for better performance and combat heat stress
- Vitamin C in the ration (150-300 gm per ton of feed) can protect birds from the effects of heat stress and enhance the survival of birds exposed to acute heat stress.
- Use vitamin and electrolyte supplements in the drinking water. Shifts in the acid/base balance in the blood of heat stressed birds cause the loss of sodium, chloride, potassium, and bicarbonate in the urine. The use of electrolyte solutions in the drinking water may help to replenish these minerals and correct the acid/base balance.
- During periods of high temperature, the flock has higher demand for drinking water. The water to feed ratio is normally 2:1 at 21°C (70°F), but increases to 4:1 at 40°C (104°F). For floor raised flocks, providing additional drinkers can help to fulfil the increased requirement

Management strategies in heat stress

- Paint the roofs with reflective material such as shiny and smooth white wash. In dry climates, apply stalking material such as straw or dry grass (at least 8 cm thick) on the roof for insulation from solar heat.
- Postpone routine management practices which require bird handling, such as eye, nasal drop vaccinations and carry out operations during the cooler parts of the day (early morning or late evening) or at night.
- Adjust the amounts of medications and volumes of water used for water vaccinations to reflect the increased water consumption of the flock during hot weather.
- Do not withhold drinking water from the flock when vaccine is provided through drinking water. Postpone these vaccinations whenever possible as heat stressed birds have decreased immune function and may not respond well to vaccination.
- Transport birds at night with low stocking density in cages to increase the ventilation around the birds.

Catching broilers for market

Catching the broiler chicken for market is the final step in a batch wise rearing of broilers. It is of two types namely manual and machine catching and, in India, only manual catching is mostly practiced.

The good catching system design will offer the following benefits,

1. Minimum number of Dead on Arrival (DOA) on market
2. Minimum number of condemned birds due to broken limbs, damage etc.,
3. Minimum live shrink (lose in live weight during transport)
4. Hygienic slaughter
5. Improved broiler welfare

Perquisites for good catching programme

1. Well trained catch crew
2. Adequate number of personnel

3. Planning in the right time – preferably evening – cooler part of the day
4. Adequate number of crates
5. Well cleaned vehicles for transport
6. Well planned feed withdrawal programme

Feed withdrawal of broilers

The feed withdrawal of broiler before slaughter is necessary in optimizing feed conversion, meat yield, live shrink and plant contamination. The purpose of feed withdrawal is to empty the digestive tract, thereby preventing ingested feed and faecal material from contaminating the carcasses during the evisceration process.

Recommended time for feed withholding is 8 hours to 12 hours, which includes pre catch feed withdrawal duration, catch time, transit time to market and holding time if any, before slaughter etc., Less than 8 hours will result in excess feed and faecal residues in the digestive tract leads minimize the feed conversion. Faecal residues cause contamination of plant equipment.

Feed withdrawal in excess of 12 hours causes the loss of intestine tensile strength, making them easy to rupture. The intestinal contents will become viscous due to the intestinal cell necrosis. This condition will cause major equipment contamination in the plant.

Water withdrawal of broilers

Do not withdraw water for broilers like feed. The water for broilers must be available to birds until the catching process starts in house. If the birds are scheduled for processing plant, well planning is highly recommended in terms of transport time, holding time etc.,

Guidelines for quality broiler catching programme:

1. Ensure the availability of clean crates for transport
2. Remove all the equipments in the house
3. Maintain reasonable stocking density based on the crates floor space (Minimum of 0.5 sq.ft per bird)
4. Catching process should be done at cooler parts of the day with minimum light availability

5. Arrange for reasonable number of bird catchers
6. Restrict movement of the birds by partition arrangements

Manual catching of broilers

The most common methods of manual catching are by the feet or by the back and mostly by the feet.

1. Grab the bird only by its shank
2. Maximum holding per hand is 4-5 birds
3. Handling birds not more than once
4. Do not pass birds between catchers.
5. Back catching is limited to 2 birds at a time

Based on the above conditions, a perfect broiler catching programme is requiring well planned schedule of activities with a stipulated time line.

Activity

1. Visit the local market and prepare a list of broiler feed ingredients available and its cost.
2. List the various litter materials available in your area and its cost.
3. Prepare feed formulae for broiler pre starter, starter and finisher feed with available feed ingredients in your area.
4. Prepare a feed formulae for broiler finisher feed for summer season.

❑❑❑

Chapter 7

Bio Security in Commercial Broiler Farm

Learning objectives:

1. *List the critical steps in quality bio security programme*
2. *Design a disinfection protocol for a commercial broiler farm*
3. *Execute a vaccination programme for a commercial broiler farm*

Concept of bio security

The concept of bio security in broiler farm facility is the collection of measures taken, to prevent the entry and attack of bio pathogens on broiler and it works on three objectives,

1. To prevent the entry of disease producing pathogens in to farm
2. To prevent the spread of disease producing organisms within the farm
3. To minimize the incidence of zoonotic health problems

In a holistic bio security plan there are three approaches and they are :

1. **Conceptual bio security**: It involves selection of bio secure site-virgin for broiler farm - topographically ideal - logistically friendly water safe, pollution free etc., for broiler farm operations- In most cases, problems in conceptual bio security cannot be over come at ease at later date, thereby it warrants careful planning.
2. **Structural bio security**: Poultry farm layout – construction buildings and sheds- distance between poultry sheds- feed mill - staff quarters - water tank- dead bird disposal plant etc., and its position related to others. Consultation with a poultry consultant is a must for this process.
3. **Operational bio security:** It consist of daily routine bio security managemental procedures like- isolation of sick birds and

quarantine of new stock-cleaning and disinfection of broiler houses-vaccination and medication-restriction of personnel entry-dead bird disposal- etc. This needs a detailed and well structured schedule of programme for a holistic approach.

General routes of pathogen transmission

1. Bird : (transfer of birds from place to place, new stock, free ranging bird, sick birds).
2. Other animals: (wild animals, domestic animals, rodents).
3. People (farm personnel, service personal, drivers, visitors).
4. Equipments (dirty equipments like feeders, drinkers, crates, egg trays and boxes, chick boxes etc.).
5. Vehicles (trucks of feed and birds lifting vehicle).
6. Air (aerosol transmission).
7. Water (contaminated water).
8. Feed (old feed and long storage feed with fungus problems).

Strategies for prevention of pathogen entry in to the farm

1. Peripheral fencing of the total farm area
2. Gate provision and gate log maintenance for visitors and vehicles
3. Provision of foot bath, truck wash, disinfection wash/shower of humans
4. Source birds from a disease-free history flock
5. Complete restriction for pet birds, pets and wild birds
6. Procuring clean feed ingredients or feed from the trusted sources
7. Systematic allocation of labours for different operations
8. Optimal down time (three weeks) between two batches

Bio security measures in dead bird disposal

1. Dead birds will attract insect, wild and domesticated animals and acting as a potential source of infection to the farm.

2. Collection of dead birds should be two times day after suitable post-mortem examination.
3. Dead birds should be handled properly by burial, incineration, composting or rendering which is based on the choice.
4. Carcass disposal trucks should be cleaner every day.
5. Bio security signs should be posted in the dead bird transport truck

Disinfection in broiler farm facility

Microbial contamination is a major cause factor for the incidence of disease. It can be prevented and controlled using proper set of management practices and that is called as disinfection and sanitation procedures and collectively called as decontamination process of broiler facilities. Decontamination process involves two steps namely *Cleaning* and *Disinfection*.

1. Cleaning is a process of physical removing dust, soil, organic matter like droppings, blood and any waste secretions from a surface and disinfection cannot be substitute of improper cleaning and a good cleaning is a base for effective disinfection. Cleaning is of two types and they are *dry cleaning* and *wet cleaning*
   a) Dry Cleaning: Brushing, scraping, etc. of inside and outside the buildings, equipments etc.,
   b) Wet Cleaning: Wet cleaning involves cleaning with detergent mixed water like soaking, washing and rinsing of surfaces and equipments.
2. Disinfection specifically denotes the use of chemicals in the cleaning process. Generally the list of chemicals used for disinfection process is based on their chemical nature,
   a) Alcohols (Ethyl alcohol and Iso propyl alcohol)
   b) Halogens (Idodophors, Chlorines)
   c) Quaternary Ammonium Compounds
   d) Phenolic compounds
   e) Aldehydes (Glutaraldehyde and Formalin)
   f) Oxidizing Agents (Hydrogen peroxide)

The choice of disinfectant for a particular process in based on number of factors and they are :

1. The cleanliness of place
2. The type of organisms in target
3. Efficacy of the disinfectant against a microorganism
4. Contact time
5. Residual activity requirements.
6. Cost
7. Human health hazard problems

For effective implementation of disinfection procedures, right choice of disinfectant is mandatory for which clear understanding of different terminologies used in this process will be helpful.

- *Sterilization* - The destruction of all infective and reproductive forms of all microorganisms (bacteria, fungi, virus, etc.).
- *Disinfection* - The destruction of all vegetative forms of microorganisms. Spores are not destroyed.
- *Sanitation* - The reduction of pathogenic organism numbers to a level at which they do not pose a disease threat to their host.

Formaldehyde gas fumigation

Fumigation with formaldehyde gas is an effective method for disinfecting the broiler house. Formaldehyde gas is commercially available as formalin (37% formaldehyde in water) or paraformaldehyde (91% formaldehyde). When either product is heated, formaldehyde gas is produced. It is quite toxic, with a tolerance of 5 ppm in air and inhalation should be avoided.

Directions for use of formalin

The heat necessary to release formaldehyde gas form formalin is best produced by mixing potassium permanganate ($KMnO_4$) with it. Use an enamelware or earthenware vessel of large capacity because of the boiling, foaming, splattering action when the two are mixed. Place the vessel in the area to be fumigated, add the permanganate first in the vessel, and then add formalin. Never add the permanganate to formalin.

Recommendations for mixing permanganate with formalin

Two parts (by volume) of formalin are mixed with approximately one part (by weight) of potassium permanganate. This will produce complete expulsion of the gas. When the reaction is complete, a dry, brown powder will be left. If the residue is wet, not enough permanganate was used; if the residue is purple, too much permanganate was used. Varying concentrations of formaldehyde gas are necessary to fumigate under different conditions. The normal or single strength concentration (1 X concentration) is obtained by mixing 40 ml of formalin with 20 g of potassium permanganate for each 100 cubic feet (2.83 cubic meter) of space. Likewise, 2 X, 3 X and 5 x concentrations are produced by respective increase in the quantity of chemicals in the same space. Empty broiler houses shall be fumigated with 3 X or 4 X concentrations for effective disinfection.

Temperature and humidity for maximum formaldehyde disinfection

For getting maximum disinfection, the optimum temperature of the area to be fumigated is 75 ^{0}F (24 ^{0}C), or higher, and the relative humidity is 75%, or more and the effective contact time is 20 minutes.

Neutralizing formaldehyde gas

In certain instances it is necessary to stop the action of formaldehyde gas after the required period of fumigation. Usually this may be accomplished by opening the air intakes and exhausts in the houses, but often this method is too slow. A solution of 27-29 per cent ammonium hydroxide (NH_4OH) solution is used to neutralize the formaldehyde gas.

Strength of formaldehyde fumigation

Varying concentrations of formaldehyde gas are needed under different conditions and the length of the fumigation period is variable. The gas is detrimental to the living embryo and to the newly hatched chick, and care must be exercised that the concentration of the gas and the length of the fumigation period meet the requirements to kill all the pathogenic organisms possible, yet not be lethal to the embryo or chick.

Methods to prevent the incidence of diseases

Vaccination

Vaccination is one of the important tools in disease prevention of broiler flock. In intensive broiler production, almost from all the viral diseases, birds are being protected through vaccination program only. It is not possible to recommend standard broiler vaccination program for all parts of country due to number of factors like, type of bird, endemicity of a disease, climate etc.

However, location specific and strategically sound vaccination programme will be helpful to prevent disease outbreak in most of the times, but, faulty vaccination will always fail to protect the birds from disease attack and sometimes it may act as source for infection. The purpose of vaccination is to improve the bird's immunity against a particular disease causing agent, thereby preventing from its pathogenic effects.

Vaccines are generally delicate products, having shorter shelf life in storage (mostly cold storage), improper handling will reduce its potency in their action. The important part of vaccination program is recommended vaccination schedule for a particular farm, which should be prepared by the experienced native poultry consultant based on their experience in his work area or the prescriptions of the veterinary institutions or breeders specifications or combination of all these. Moreover, any vaccination program should be carried out under the supervision of qualified veterinary consultant.

Types of vaccine

Live vaccine - the active part of the vaccine is the live organism that causes the disease. As such, it is capable of inducing the disease in birds that have not had previous contact to that organism. Cross infection can also occur.

Attenuated vaccine - with this type of vaccine the organism has been attenuated by special procedures during manufacture, so that it has lost its ability to cause the serious form of the disease but, however, the vaccine still has the ability to trigger the immune system to produce antibodies.

Killed vaccine - with this type of vaccine the organism has been killed and is unable to cause the disease, although the ability to trigger the immune system remains.

Vaccine forms

1. Liquid vaccine – it is in fluid form ready to use.
2. Freeze dried vaccine – the vaccine stored in freeze dried form for longer shelf life and it should be reconstituted with diluents before use.

Common vaccination methods in broiler farm

There are a number of methods of vaccination available; the choice of particular methods depends on vaccine and its type. In some of the methods that individual vaccination has to be carried out and in some other, mass vaccination can be followed.

1. Ocular Route: This method involves the vaccine being put into one of the bird's eyes by a dropper. The vaccine makes its way into the respiratory tract via the lacrimal duct. The vaccine is delivered through an eyedropper and care must be taken to ensure that the dropper delivers the recommended dose.
2. Nasal Route: This method involves introducing the vaccine into the birds' nostrils either as a dust or as a drop and closing of one nasal orifice will make the bird to suck the vaccine inside immediately.
3. Drinking water: In this method, vaccine is mixed with water and administered as regular drinking water and it less time consuming and less stressful. All equipment used for vaccination is carefully cleaned and free of detergents and disinfectants. Only cold, clean water of drinking quality should be used. Before vaccination, birds should be water starved for some time to increase the thirst and proper intake of vaccination dose through water.
4. Subcutaneous injection: This method is similar intramuscular injection but vaccine is injected under the loose skin (back of the neck) and care must be taken to ensure that the vaccine is injected into the bird and not just into the feathers or fluff in the case of very young chickens.
5. Intramuscular injection: This method involves the use of a hypodermic needle to inject the vaccine into the muscle (breast / thigh muscle) of the bird and nowadays automatic vaccinators available for maintaining accuracy of dose and ease in management and it needs some amount of training.

However, in commercial broiler farming operations, ocular and nasal route methods are widely employed for live vaccines along with drinking water method.

General guidelines for proper vaccination programme

1. Procure vaccine from standard companies, which maintain quality standards in production and cold storage in supply chain
2. Vaccination should be done at the cooler parts of the day (Morning or Evening)
3. Check the expiry date
4. Read the instructions carefully on the label of the vaccine pack
5. Exact dose of administration (extra label dose should be avoided)
6. Vaccination should not be done during disease or stress conditions
7. Very young chicks should not be vaccinated- maternal antibodies may interfere the immune response
8. Equipment used for vaccination should be cleaned and sterilised
9. Vaccination should be done by trained personnel under veterinarian supervision

General guidelines for live viral vaccines programmes

1. Live vaccines should always be kept in a refrigerator or in a freezer
2. Reconstitute the vaccine 2 hours before its use and should not kept unused for longer time
3. Cool the diluents to 4-6°C before making dilution
4. Take small amount of vaccine in a dropper, so as to utilize it within 20 minutes
5. Empty vaccine and vaccine containers should be incinerated or deep buried.
6. Vaccination should be one go programme without any time gaps

General guidelines for vaccination through drinking water

In intensive broiler production environments, taking individual bird for vaccination is a time consuming process and vaccination through drinking water is easy vaccination procedure however, it is having some limitations that ensuring the dose take up by individual bird cannot be ascertained. Moreover, primary vaccinations cannot be done through drinking water and it is highly suitable for secondary (booster) vaccinations. Considering that, following are the list of precautions to be taken during drinking water vaccinations.

1. All drinkers, utensils and pipelines used for vaccinations should be cleaned with non-medicated water
2. Drinking water to be used for vaccine preparation should not contain any detergents or medicines that may kill the organisms in vaccine.
3. Water should be cooled by adding ice, and skimmed milk powder may be used at 5 gm per litre of water as a stabilizer of the virus in the vaccine
4. Birds should be made thirsty by withdrawing water for about two hours before vaccination.
5. Vaccine should be mixed in a quantity of water (10-15 % of the total water intake per day) that it would be utilised by birds within two hours.
6. Ensure every bird is taking sufficient water there by taking prescribed dose of vaccine.
7. Birds should not be disturbed during the vaccination process.

Common vaccination schedule for broiler chicken

S.No	Age	Vaccine	Route of administration
1	5-7th day	Newcastle disease vaccine (F strain - Preferable)	Ocular / Nasal drop
2	14th day	IBD vaccine	Ocular / Nasal drop
3	21st day	Newcastle disease vaccine (Lasota strain - Preferable)	Ocular / Nasal drop

Entrepreneur / promoter should consult a poultry consultant / technical managers of breeder companies for structured programme for their flock One drop is equal to 30 micro litre*

Methods of broiler carcass disposal

Dead birds in poultry farm are potential source pathogens for causing disease spread with in the farm and outside the farm.

Considering this problem, utmost care should be taken to dispose the dead birds effectively. Collection of carcass should be carried out twice a day and on the day itself it should be disposed scientifically. There are number of ways to dispose the carcass and each method is having merits and demerits. Considering, size of operation, cost and its effectiveness, suitable methods can be selected and implemented.

Methods of broiler carcass disposal

1 *Burial in pits*	i. Burial pits are simple, convenient, inexpensive disposal method.
	ii. Burial pit site should be away (Minimum 50 m) from, broiler sheds, drinking water sources and human residences.
	iii. Pits should be constructed on well-drained sites with a compact subsoil or with a lining of clay in lose sub soil to minimize the seepage and environmental pollution
	iv. Well designed disposal pit of 5 x 2 x 3 m (30 m^3) should be sufficient to handle carcasses from a 10,000 broiler chicken farm for two years, assuming a normal mortality of 5-7 per cent per batch.
	v. Opening of 20 cm in diameter has to provided for dumping the birds
2 *Tank disposal*	i. Electrically heated tank is a operated to dispose the carcass
	ii. Safe but expensive
	iii. Digesting the carcass at the heat of around 40°C for 15 days
	iv. System depends on the activity of mesophilic bacteria accelerating decomposition.
3 *Burning*	i. Burning is the most effective and complete way of destroying infectious material.
	ii. Smokeless and odourless incinerators are available for the disposal of broiler carcasses.
	iii. Position of incinerators should be placed downwind of both broiler houses and human residences
	iv. Carcasses must be reduced to a completely burnt white ash

	v. Capital investment, fuel cost and existing regulations in a particular locality are the main considerations
4 *Rendering*	i. Rendering is the most scientific method of converting broiler carcasses into a valuable, biologically-safe protein by-product meal. ii. Rendering is defined as a process of using high temperature and pressure to convert whole animal and poultry carcasses or their by-products with no or very low value to safe, nutritional, and economically valuable products. iii. Transport of broiler carcass to central facility is a additional process in large scale rendering and cost intensive iv. Bio security of rendering plant site is critical v. The rendering temperature of (130-140^0 C) for 20-30 minutes is sufficient disinfection and even sterilization vi. Highly suitable for large operations with centralized rendering process facility
5 *Compost*	i. Composting is a controlled, natural process in which beneficial microorganisms (bacteria and fungi) reduce and transform organic waste into a useful end-product (termed compost). ii. Composting broiler carcasses provides an economical and biologically safe means of converting carcass into an odourless, humus-like material which is useful as a soil amendment and a source of plant nutrients iii. Use of composting in commercial broiler operations is very minimal

Activity

1. List the commercial vaccines available for broiler chicken in market
2. Visit a commercial broiler farm in your area and record the vaccination schedule
3. Visit a broiler processing plant and document the carcass disposal system
4. Design a fumigation schedule for broiler house with 200 ft length and 25 ft width dimensions.

❑❑❑

Chapter 8

Good Husbandry Practices and Broiler Welfare

Learning Objectives:

1. *Discuss the role of Good Husbandry Practices in broiler welfare*
2. *Identification of critical areas for implementation of GHP to improve broiler welfare*

Definition of Good Husbandry Practices in broiler farming

Good Husbandry Practices (GHP) in broiler farming can be defined as a collection of package of practices to be followed in intensive or industrial broiler production systems to maximize/optimize the production and productivity without compromising the reasonable broiler welfare.

However, Good Husbandry Practices is not a new set of practices of growing or production methods, but they are all *refined or improved* methods of our regular production activities in the production process, to achieve the overall goodness in the production to market value chain.

Benefits of GHP in broiler production value chain

Application of Good Husbandry Practices in broiler production will offer the following benefits to the broiler producer and consumer.

- Maximization of production and productivity
- Optimization of return per unit investment
- Food safety
- Improved broiler welfare
- Improved marketability of the products
- Satisfaction of producer and consumer

What is the special need for GHP in broiler farming?

Globally, broiler production is characterized by intensive rearing systems. Nowadays, in all the intensive system of broiler production, broiler welfare, and pollution are becoming the issues of discussion, more than maximizing the production and productivity.

Though, we get maximum production benefits in the intensive system of broiler production, the welfare and pollution are very serious issues to be taken care of by producers (often neglected) for a holistic, humane and sustainable production environments.

Here, it is worthy to mention that in industrial broiler production, since the capital input is very high, there is every possibility of providing inhumane treatment to animals, callous attitude towards chicken welfare and pollution.

It is the right time to sensitize the stakeholders of this production environment about the Good Husbandry Practices to be followed in intensive production systems to maximize the productivity with *improved welfare* to broiler chicken.

Broiler welfare

As per the dictionary (Oxford / Webster) references, welfare associates with state of well being, health, happiness and successful progress in life, which may rightly suits for human welfare. However, the definition of health, happiness and progress is a highly subjective term in human life, which is based on individualistic culture and priorities.

Application of the same context in the area of broiler welfare may not be right and logical, since these broiler chickens (birds of specific production function for human use) have specific and pre determined purposes for their living.

Based on that, we may not be in a comfortable position to account the "happiness factors" in animal welfare, because often they are not directly measurable and some times over ride by the production function.

Considering these background, it is reasonable to take up the definition of animal welfare proposed by World Organisation for Animal Health (OIE) that is *"how well an animal is able to cope with the conditions in which it lives"*, though, this definition lacks complete acceptance from animal welfare activists.

The reasons for the lack of acceptance of this definition is, it does not accounting the criticality of animal's feelings and experiences like happiness or stress factors. However, considering the perspective of Good Husbandry Practices in broiler farming, the definition of OIE will holds good to achieve the purpose, because OIE opined that good housing, feeding, management, disease prevention, humane handling and slaughter are the mandatory factors for a holistic broiler welfare programme.

Principles of animal welfare

Describing and assessing the broiler welfare in intensive broiler production environments is complex and often debatable. In a holistic view, broiler welfare is based on various components and can be broadly classified in to two namely effective performance of production function (meat production) and other factors like happiness, freedom to lead natural way of life of its own etc.,

For an example, a hybrid commercial broiler can gain weight of 2.2 kg in six week of period indicates that, it is that it is in clear state of well being, because of that only, it can able to produce such performance.

However, in other way, it may need not be at welfare state considering its limitations in its freedom as fowl to move in a range land. Therefore, it is important to be able to measure each component of welfare independently and integrating the different measures to reach an overall conclusion about welfare status. However, there are some guiding principles are available based on various research works to assess the overall welfare quality and they are called as Five Freedom approach in animal welfare.

The Five freedoms, principles and criteria for good animal welfare

United Kingdom's farm animal welfare council proposed that, all farm animals should have five freedoms to ensure minimum welfare environments in their rearing systems and they are freedom from,

1. Hunger and thirst
2. Discomfort

3. Pain, injury and disease
4. Express normal behaviour
5. Fear and distress

The reason for accepting welfare definition of OIE in *Good Husbandry Practices in broiler* is, OIE considers these five freedom approach as guiding principles for providing welfare to the broiler chicken and, it also being endorsed by most of the European welfare legislations and forms the basis for OIE Terrestrial Animal Health Code.

However, there is different school of thought that, it is very difficult to find out the natural behaviour of an animal in captive environments and in most cases adaptation will become a overriding factor in expression of normal behaviour, thereby problems in assessing the overall welfare quality- For an example, though *wing flapping* is normal behaviour, caged hens wing flaps occasionally due to adaptation

European Welfare Quality Consortium improved this approach and suggested guiding principles and criteria for animal welfare quality as follows,

Welfare principles	Welfare criteria (measures)
Good feeding	1. Absence of prolonged hunger (feeding space)
	2. Absence of prolonged thirst (drinker space and quantity of water intake)
Good housing	3. Comfort around resting (cleanliness and litter quality)
	4. Thermal comfort (panting and huddling)
	5. Ease of movement (stocking density)
Good health	6. Absence of pain
	7. Absence of Injuries (lameness, hock burn, foot pad dermatitis)
	8. Absence of Disease (mortality, culled outs, production performances)
Animal Behaviour	9. Expression of social and other behaviours
	10. Good human animal relationship (Avoidance Distance Test- ADT)
	11. Positive emotional state (Quality Behavior Assessment-QBA)

Assessment of broiler welfare

The scientific assessment of broiler welfare is usually a complex process, which is based on number of parameters. It includes a range of physical, physiological, behavioural or clinical indicators, and comparing these measurements among chickens that are reared in a specific production system. A broad range of indicators can be used to assess stress response and immune function in an attempt to measure whether the animal is coping with its environment or not. However, interpretation of these indicators is sometimes difficult. The measures of welfare can be classified in to two namely,

Resource based measure for broilers	Animal based measure for broilers
1. Stocking density	1. Livability / Mortality
2. Feeder and Drinker space	2. Per cent culled
3. No. of feeders and drinkers	3. Lameness
4. Micro environment	4. Hock burn
(temperature and relative humidity	5. Injuries of birds
5. Air quality (ammonia)	6. Food pad dermatitis
6. Litter quality	7. Human relationship (Avoidance
(moisture & freshness)	Distance Test)
	8. Quality Behaviour Assessment

However, conventionally we used to think that optimization of resource based measure will ensure welfare, but it is not necessarily always. Combination of these two measures of welfare will provide picture about the actual status of welfare in production environment.

In intensive broiler production systems, interaction between welfare and production goals is *bi directionally associated* (positive or negative), which is based on the specific production function and goal and they can be explained as follows,

1. Improved methods of feeding, disease prevention (welfare measures) will ensure the welfare of broiler and lead to high production gains, in which, welfare and production is positively associated.
2. Restricting feed intake in broiler breeder chicken will avoid the over eating and excess body weight, improve the uniformity for

the prescribed body weights at the specific ages, in turn improve the production function (hatching egg production), but it may be a factor for chronic hunger (against welfare) for these birds. In this situation production gain and welfare are negatively associated.

When production gains can be achieved by improving animal welfare, there is be no need for any safe-guard mechanism for broiler welfare, because of its dual benefits. However, when increased production gains, conflicts with welfare, some mechanisms are required to ensure a *reasonable* welfare with human touch. In these circumstances, how to ensure reasonable welfare without compromising production and productivity is a challenging situation, in which application Good Husbandry Practices will be a useful strategy and it shall be made available in the form of law, codes of practice and voluntary welfare assurance programs etc.

Welfare issues in commercial broiler production

Identification of welfare issues in intensive broiler production is a basic process to implement Good Husbandry Practices, and to improve the welfare. Following are the list of indicative welfare issues in intensive broiler production environment.

Indicative List of welfare issues in commercial broiler farming systems

Broiler	Transport of broiler day old chicks
	Vaccination at day old
	Brooder management
	Over crowding
	Lack of adequate heat
	Starvation during brooding
	Lack of good quality litter and desirable moisture
	Improper micro environment
	Poor air quality in broiler houses
	Poor quality feed
	Poor quality water
	Lack of optimum feeding and drinking space
	Frequent vaccination and medication
	Feed withdrawal time before slaughter
	Catching and transport of birds for market
	Skeletal problems (foot pad dermatitis/hock burn)
	Culled broilers (unfit for slaughter)

Benefits of GHP and welfare

Implementation Good Husbandry Practices in broiler farming offers benefits in three forms namely, improved production and consumer acceptance, wide access to markets and creation of employment. Growing awareness on welfare issues of in intensive broiler farming among the consumers of broiler chicken products, make the people to choose products from chicken raised in good welfare conditions, which leads improved acceptance of those products without any hesitation, thereby providing satisfaction to producer and consumer.

Activity

1. Visit a commercial broiler farm and take a account of the resource based measure in assessing the broiler welfare.
2. Compare two commercial broiler farm's welfare by calculating the realized stocking density.
3. Compare two broiler farms in terms of incidence of food pad dermatitis while lifting the birds for market or processing plants.

❑❑❑

Chapter 9

Performance Indices in Broiler Chicken Farming

Learning Objectives:

1. *List out the economic traits of commercial broiler*
2. *Work out production performance indices for commercial broiler farms*

In broiler farming system, a trait (character) can be defined as any measurable attribute of phenotype/production function with respect its quality and quantity of production. Economic traits are traits, which are having significant economic importance, there by influencing the economics of production function.

Understanding the concept and application of economic traits in production performance analysis is a key factor, for any farm manager, when optimizing the cost economics, especially when welfare and production function interests are having bi directional association.

Economic traits of chicken broiler

S.No.	Economic Traits
1.	Hatch weight – Weight of day old broiler chick at the time of hatch after complete drying.
2.	Body weight at first, second, third, fourth, fifth, sixth weeks and up to market age.
3.	Feed consumption up to first, second, third, fourth, fifth, sixth weeks and up to market age.
4.	i) Live body weight gain – Differences in body weights between two periods. ii) Average Daily Gain (ADG) - Mean daily body weight gain during a period of grow out.

5. i) Feed Efficiency or Feed Conversion Ratio (FCR) – Quantity of feed consumption per unit of live body weight gain.

   ii) Period wise Feed Conversion Efficiency - Calculated for period wise as Quantity of feed consumption in period interval / Weight gain in a period interval (Eg. fourth week feed efficiency)

   iii) Cumulative Feed Conversion Efficiency- Quantity of feed consumption up to a period / Weight gain up to a period (Eg. feed efficiency up to fourth week)

6. Market age (number of days of grow for a broiler to reach the market weight)

7. Livability / Mortality (live / death) expressed in percent

   a) Brooding period (up to three weeks)

   b) Growing period (four weeks to market age)

   c) Overall mortality up to market age

8. i) Live shrink (per cent live weight loss from point of catching to point of market or processing plant)

   ii) Per cent DOA – Dead on Arrival (mortality during catching and transit to the retail outlets or processing plant)

9. i) Dressing yield (carcass yield after blood and feather loss)

   ii) Eviscerated yield (carcass yield after evisceration)

   iii) Ready to cook yield (eviscerated yield plus giblets (heart, liver, gizzard yield)

   iv) Condemned carcass

   v) Breast meat yield

   vi) All the traits are conventionally expressed in per cent

Broiler Performance Efficiency Factor (BPEF)

Broiler Performance Efficiency Factor is a comprehensive tool to assess and compare the performance of two batches of broilers or strains in holistic manner and it depends on production performance measures namely,

1. Live market weight
2. Market age
3. Feed Conversion Efficiency
4. Livability

BPEF can be calculated using the following formulae and the values above 300 will be of optimum for commercial broiler strains.

$$\frac{\text{Liveweight (kg)} \times \text{Livability (\%)}}{\text{Market age (days)} \times \text{Feed Conversion Efficiency}} \times 100$$

Broiler performance calculation

Calculation of production indices (on batch wise)

In commercial broiler farming, the critical production indices are,

1. Mean live market weight
2. Mean market age
3. Feed Conversion Ratio
4. Livability
5. Cost of feed per broiler
6. Broiler Performance Efficiency Factor

All these performances are dependent on number of factors like commercial strain, system of rearing, feeding and management protocols, health conditions of the bird etc.

Example:

In a commercial broiler farm, the following data were recorded for a batch of broilers.

1.	Total floor space	:	12,000 sq.ft
2.	Day old chick placement	:	10,500 Nos.
3.	Age of lifting of broiler for market	:	39 days
4.	Mortality	:	475 Nos.
5.	Total live broilers lifted for market	:	10,025 Nos.
6.	Total live weight output	:	21,854 kg
7.	Total feed intake	:	38,244 kg
8.	Average cost of feed	:	Rs. 30 per kg

Computation of batch production indices

1	Mean Market weight	Total live weight output divide by Number of birds lifted for market (21854 kg/10025 Nos.)	2.18 kg
2	Mean market age	Actual Note: If the birds are lifted in various days, workout the average of the same	39 days
3	Livability	100 – (Number of birds died divide by total number of birds housed *100)	95.47 %
4	Batch FCR	Total quantity of feed consumption in kg divide by Total live broiler output in kg(38244 /21854)	1.75
5	Feed cost per broiler	Mean market weight (kg) x Feed Conversion Ratio x Average cost of feed per kg (2.18 x 1.75 x 30 x)	Rs.114.45
6	BPEF	$\frac{\text{(Liveweight (kg) x Livability (\%))}}{\text{(Market age (days) x Feed Conversion Efficiency)}} \times 100$ $\frac{\text{(2.18 (kg) x 95.47 (\%))}}{\text{(39 days x 1.75)}} \times 100$	305

Activity

In a commercial broiler farm, the following data were recorded for a batch of broilers.

1.	Total floor space	: 20,000 sq.ft
2.	Day old chick placement	: 19,500Nos.
3.	Age of lifting of broiler for market	: 40 days
4.	Mortality	: 625 Nos.
5.	Total live broilers lifted for market	: 18,875 Nos.
6.	Total live weight output	: 41713 kg
7.	Total feed intake	: 72,164 kg
8.	Average cost of feed	: Rs. 30.50

Calculate the following and offer your comments.

1. Mean market weight of broiler
2. Stocking density
3. Mean market age

4. Livability
5. Feed efficiency
6. Cost of feed per broiler
7. Cost of feed per kg live weight
8. Broiler Performance Efficiency Factor

Fill up the blank cells in the table

Age (week)	Body weight(g)	Weekly Gain (g)	Cumulative gain(g)	Feed consumption (g)		Feed Conversion		Avg. daily-feed intake (g)	Avg. Daily Gain (g)
				Weekly (g)	Cumulative (g)	Weekly (g)	Cumulative (g)		
1	180			145					
2	442			320					
3	815			510					
4	1270			758					
5	1795			1028					
6	2395			1330					

Hatch weight: 41 gram

❑❑❑

Chapter 10

Economics of a Commercial Broiler Farm

Learning Objectives:

1. *Discuss the cost of production of broiler chicken*
2. *Prepare of a project report for a commercial broiler farm*

Understanding the economics of a commercial broiler farm is a final step in the learning process about the subject of commercial broiler production. It will be helpful for financial planning of broiler farm and to prepare a project report for availing financial assistance from the banks.

The cost of production in broiler farming implies, the total cost of production of broiler chicken on unit basis or live weight basis, which includes primarily feed cost, chick cost, labour cost, other over heads etc., However, in financial parlance cost may classified in to three namely fixed investment, fixed cost and variable cost. Understanding these costs will helpful to work out economics in a proper way.

Fixed investment

Fixed investment is the investment made by the promoter or entrepreneur to develop the broiler farm facilities, which includes, purchase of land, land preparation, construction of broiler houses, equipments, facilities for water and accessories like office, quarters, godown and outlet if any etc. Generally, in fixed investment, 75 per cent will be provided by the financial institutions and 25 per cent will be borne by the promoter.

Fixed cost

Fixed cost is the cost, fixed in nature and does not vary with volume of production. Cost on fixed investment in the form of interest and depreciation on building and equipments value (assumed cost) are come under fixed cost.

Variable cost

Variable cost is the cost, variable in nature and, will vary with the volume of production. Chick, feed, labour, electricity, litter, health management inputs, other utilities and over heads will come under the variable cost.

Total cost

Total cost is the cost which includes fixed and variable cost

Economics of commercial broiler chicken farm depends on four factors for its profitability and they are,

1. **Broiler farm size :** Volume of production favours the cost economics and it is called as " economy of scale " and cost of production per unit will be minimum.
2. **Cost of inputs :** Low cost of inputs favours the economics positively.
3. **Realized technical performance of the farm**: Realized technical performance indicates the performance of broiler farm in their economic traits like live body weight, feed efficiency, mortality etc., and its overall performance.
4. **Sale price of outputs:** High sale price of the output favours the economics positively.

Model economics of a commercial broiler chicken farm

Broiler farm size

1. Independent / own farm type
2. Broiler farm size : 20,000 broiler per batch
3. All in All out system of rearing
4. Deep litter system of housing

Technical Standards: Technical standards are the assumed/ expected performance of a commercial broiler farm under certain pre conditions and assumptions. It should be on par with the average industry standards.

1	Cost of land - Nil	: Farmer's own land
2	Cost of land preparation	: Rs. 2,00,000/-
3	Cost of construction of deep litter broiler houses	: Rs. 140 per sq.ft
4	Floor space requirement	: 1 sq.ft per bird
5	Cost of equipments and other accessories	: Rs. 20 per bird
6	Down time (time gap between two batches)	: 3 weeks
7	Average number of batches expected to grown	: 5 batches per year
8	Cost of day old chick	: Rs. 20 per chick
9	Cost of feed	: Rs. 30 per kg
10	Cost vaccination and medication and other utilities	: Rs. 5 per bird
11	Labour cost	: Rs. 8 per bird
12	Mean market age	: 42 days
13	Mean live weight	: 2.25 kg
14	Mean feed conversion ratio	: 1.75
15	Livability	: 95 per cent
16	Sale price on live weight basis	: Rs.85 per kg
17	Interest on investment	: 15 % pa
18	Depreciation on building	: 10 % pa
19	Depreciation on equipments	: 15 % pa

Economics (for a year)

S. No.	Items	Amount (Rs.)
A.	**Fixed investment**	
A1	Cost of Land	: Nil
A2	Cost of preparation of land of broiler farm	: 2,00,000
A3	Cost of construction of broiler houses [20,000 x 1(sq.ft) x Rs.140 per sq.ft]	: 28,00,000
A4	Cost of purchase of equipments and accessories [20,000 x Rs.20 per bird]	: 4,00,000
A5	**Total**	**: 34,00,000**
B.	**Fixed cost**	
B1	Cost / Interest on investment @ 15 % per annum [Rs.34,00,000 x 0.15]	: 5,10,000

B2	Depreciation on building @ 10 % per annum	: 2,80,000
B3	Depreciation on equipments @ 15 % annum	: 60,000
B4	**Total**	: **8,50,000**
C.	**Variable cost**	
C1	Cost of day old chick[20,000 x 5 batches x Rs.20 per chick]	: 20,00,000
C2	Cost of feed[20,000 x 5 (batches) 2.25 (L.wt) x 1.75 (FCR) x Rs.30]	1,18,12,500
C3	Cost of medicines, vaccines and other utilities [20,000 x 5 (batches) x Rs.5]	: 5,00,000
C4	Cost of labour [20,000 x 5 (batches) x Rs. 8]	: 8,00,000
C5	**Total**	: **1,51,12,500**
D.	**Total cost** [B plus C]	: **1,59,62,500**
E.	**Income/Receipts**	
E1	Sale of broiler chicken[20,000 x 5 (batches) x 0.95 (livability) x 2.25 (L.wt) x Rs.85 (Sale price)	: **1,81,68,750**
E2	**Gross income**	: **1,81,68,750**
E3	**Net income** [E minus D]	: **22,06,250**
E4	Net income per broiler [E3 divide by (20,000 x 5 x 0.95)]	: 23.22
E5	Cost of production per broiler [D divide by (20,000 x 5 x 0.95)]	: 168.02
E6	Benefit Cost Ratio – BCR [E divide by D]	: 1.13

Activity

Prepare a report on economics of broiler farm with a batch size of 30,000 broilers for a year using average industry technical standards.

❑❑❑

Chapter 11

References

1. Animal Welfare Approved Standards for Meat Chickens PS53v1 Meat chicken standards 2015 072715:http://animalwelfareapproved.org/wp-content/uploads/2015/10/Meat-chicken-standards-2015-v1.pdf.
2. Commercial Chicken Meat and Egg Production (2002), Fifth Edition Edited by DONALD D. BELL and WILLIAM D. WEAVER, Published by Kluwer Academic Publishers.
3. Poultry breeding and Genetics (1990).R.D.Crawford (Editor), 3rd Revised Edition, Elsevier Publications.

❑❑❑

Chapter 12

Annexures

Annexure -1

Metric conversions

Length	
1 meter	100 cm
1 meter	3.28 ft
1 feet	12 inches
1 inch	2.54 centimetres
Area	
1 hectare	2.47 acres
1 acre	4048 square meters
1 square meter	10.76 square feet
1 square feet	144 square inches
1 square feet	929 square centimetres
Area of circle	Pi r square
Weight	
1 kilo gram	2.20 pounds
1 pound	0.45 kilograms
Temperature	
Centigrade to Fahrenheit	^{o}C x 1.8 plus 32
Fahrenheit to Centigrade	(^{o}F minus 32) / by 1.8

Annexure-2

Answer key

Chapter -3	1. 67,142 sq.ft and 58,750 sq.ft 2. 1,65,600 sq.ft and 1,38,000 sq.ft
Chapter -4	1. 18.15 kg per square meter and 1.2 sq.ft per bird
Chapter -9	1. Mean market weight of broiler :2.20 kg
	2. Stocking density: 22.44 kg/square meter
	3. Mean market age: 40 days
	4. Livability:96.79 per cent
	5. Feed efficiency : 1.73. Cost of feed per broiler: Rs.116.108. Cost of feed per kg live weight: Rs.52.77. Broiler Performance Efficiency Factor: 307

❑❑❑